RELEASED

HEALTH POLICY IN THE UNITED STATES: Issues and Options

By Lawrence D. Brown

Occasional Paper Number Four
Ford Foundation Project on
Social Welfare and the American Future

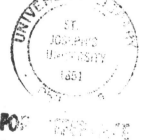
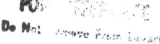

Ford Foundation
New York, N.Y.

One of a series of reports on activities by the Ford Foundation. A complete list of publications may be obtained from the Ford Foundation, Office of Reports, 320 East 43 Street, New York, New York 10017.

Health Policy in the United States: Issues and Options originated as a paper presented in November 1985 at a conference on health-care policy options convened by the New York Academy of Medicine and funded by the Ford Foundation and the United Hospital Fund of New York. It was subsequently published as an article in the *Bulletin of the New York Academy of Medicine,* Vol. 63, No. 5, June 1987. It is reprinted here in a slightly revised form with the *Bulletin*'s permission. The author wishes to thank Martin Klein for his assistance in the revisions.

Lawrence D. Brown is professor and head of the Division of Health Administration, School of Public Health, Columbia University. Formerly he was a professor in the Department of Health Services Management and Policy at the University of Michigan and a member of the Government Studies Program at the Brookings Institution. Professor Brown is author of numerous articles and books on federal health-care policy, and is the editor of the *Journal of Health Politics, Policy and Law*.

Library of Congress Cataloging-in-Publication Data
Brown, Lawrence D. (Lawrence David), 1947-
    Health Policy in the United States.
    (Occasional paper/Ford Foundation Project on Social Welfare and the American Future; no. 4)
    Includes bibliographical references.
    1. Medical policy—United States.   I. Title.   II. Series: Occasional paper (Ford Foundation. Project on Social Welfare and the American Future); no. 4
[DNLM: 1. Health Policy—United States.   WA 525 B878h]
RA395.A3B775   1988   362.1'0973   88-24413
ISBN 0-916584-34-8

467   September 1988

Cover Photograph: Abraham Menashe

EXECUTIVE PANEL
Ford Foundation Project on Social Welfare and the American Future

Contents

Foreword

The United States has a two-pronged system of social welfare—one designed for labor-force participants and the other for those who do not work in the paid labor force. For workers, a combination of employee benefit and government social insurance programs provides protection against the risks of illness, disability, and unemployment and also sets aside funds for income maintenance and health coverage during the retirement years. Nonworkers, mainly children, the disabled, and the elderly, are sustained by a governmental safety-net program. Except for low-income single parents with young children, able-bodied, working-age adults are expected to work and thereby provide for their needs.

Does this social welfare system, designed in large part in the 1930s, provide sufficient protection for Americans as they are about to enter the twenty-first century? Have significant holes developed in the fabric of social protection, and, if so, is society willing to pay for mending them? Has the changing composition of the U.S. population, specifically the increase in the elderly and single-parent families, altered the premises on which the system was built? Why is there such a persistently high level of poverty, in good times and bad, and can anything be done to correct it? Can more be done to help the troubling number of American children who experience at least some poverty in their growing-up years?

These are some of the questions that the Ford Foundation set out to answer when in 1985 it launched a wide-ranging inquiry into alternative approaches to providing social insurance and welfare services, taking into account changes in the economy, in the family and work, and in the nation's age profile. Called the Project on Social Welfare and the American Future, the inquiry is led by a twelve-member executive panel of citizens representing the business, academic, civil rights, and labor communities.* Chairman of the panel is Irving S. Shapiro, a former member of the Foundation's Board of Trustees and a former chief executive officer of the du Pont Company.

In the course of its inquiry, the panel commissioned a number of research reports and convened sessions of social policy experts to discuss approaches to such interrelated topics as health care, retirement and pension policy, poverty and welfare policy, and public and private social welfare programs. For one of the sessions, in September 1986, the panel invited leading scholars and practitioners in the field of poverty and welfare to discuss the policy implications of their work. They were asked to address three topics: the diverse and interrelated causes of poverty, the consequences of poverty for individuals and society as a whole, and whether the safety-net and training programs developed since the 1930s are appropriate for fighting poverty in the 1980s and beyond.

The reports offer an unusually comprehensive picture of why people are poor and what has been and might be done about it. For this reason, the Foundation has decided to publish them. The first two, issued in November 1987, were David T. Ellwood's review of our various income-maintenance programs and Judith M. Gueron's paper on how the welfare system might be reformed. A paper by Gordon Berlin and Andrew Sum, published in February 1988, analyzed the links between inadequate basic skills and a variety of social problems, from dropping out of school to unemployment to welfare dependency. Now Lawrence D. Brown reviews U.S. health-care policy over the past forty years and discusses ways to make health care more accessible and affordable for larger numbers. The views expressed in the papers are the authors' own and do not necessarily reflect those of members of the executive panel or of the staff and board of the Ford Foundation.

We are grateful to the authors for taking time out from their busy schedules to set down their thoughts on a range of complex issues. Together, they have made a useful contribution to the current debate over social welfare policy.

Franklin A. Thomas
President
Ford Foundation

---

* Members of the panel are listed on page iii.

Health Policy in
the United States

Introduction

To an attentive observer all periods are ones "of transition," and the sources and import of change are seldom evident except in retrospect. Even the most present-oriented student of American health policy, however, cannot fail to notice changes today that are remarkably deep and quick. Indeed, the policy picture recalls Henry Adams's impressions at the dawn of the twentieth century—"a far faster universe, where all the old roads ran about in every direction, overrunning, dividing, subdividing, stopping abruptly, vanishing slowly, with side-paths that led nowhere, and sequences that could not be proved."[1] This paper sketches the evolution of recent American health-care policy and tries to make both analytical and practical sense of it. What follows is a broad and synthetic overview of where we came from, where we now stand, and, above all, what plausible options are available for the future.

Here *policy* will be understood to mean measures that government (that is, the public sector) can adopt to advance given ends. *Ends* are desired states of the world or outcomes. They are *given* by the political process, which is presumed to reflect with some degree of fidelity society's values and preferences. *Measures* mainly means government *programs* (although moral exhortation, threats, and the like also fall into the category). And to say that government *can* adopt measures means that adopting them lies in fact within government's power, which excludes ideal but utopian policies from consideration here. A policy *issue* is a subject of concern and debate among participants in the political process. A policy *option* is someone's would-be *program*.

Defined in this way, policy comprises a vast realm of concerns, possibilities, and commitments. The subject cannot be examined productively until some analytical categories have been imposed on it. My approach groups programs by the ends and strategies of governmental intervention, that is, by the policy types they represent.

Broadly speaking, the United States federal government (and for that matter central governments in most other comparable countries) intervenes in the health-care system with four objectives in mind, and uses four main policy strategies to achieve them. First, government may want to influence the *supply* of health-care services and resources, especially the stock of biomedical research, technology, hospitals, and personnel. In the United States this goal has been advanced largely by extending federal grants to providers (broadly defined) to augment their continuing activities or to innovate. This *subsidy* strategy has taken the programmatic form of grants to the National Institutes of Health, the Hill-Burton program, and various programs assisting medical schools and medical students.

Second, government may want to influence the *demand* for health care among all or part of the population. The usual expression of this *financing* strategy is a health insurance program, created under public auspices and financed in whole or part by public funds, that helps consumers to pay all or part of their medical bills. The European norm is universal national health insurance; in the United States the major programs are Medicare (for the old, the disabled, and those in need of renal dialysis) and Medicaid (for the welfare poor and medically indigent).

Third, government may want to alter the *organization* of the health-care system by building new organizations to serve special subgroups in the population (for instance, the Veterans Administration health-care system, Community Health Centers, the National Health Service Corps) or to advance some larger goal (for example, health maintenance organizations and other "alternative delivery systems" intended to help society as a whole to contain health costs). The strategy, then, is *reorganization*.

Fourth, government may want to influence the *behavior* of providers, especially with respect to the use, price, and quality of services, and the size, location, and equipment of facilities. Major *regulatory* programs include the Professional Standards Review Organizations, transformed in 1982 into Peer Review Organizations; planning by means of Comprehensive Health Planning Agencies, and, later, Health Systems Agencies; setting of prospective hospital rates in such states as New Jersey, Maryland, and New York, and by the Prospective Payment

System adopted by the federal government in 1983 for inpatient services in Medicare; and capital expenditures review under section 1122 of the Social Security Amendments of 1972 and state certificate-of-need programs.

In the United States these strategies have emerged in roughly chronological sequence, the later ones intended in part to address and correct the problems of those that preceded. The subsidy strategy, the first flower of the new federal activism in health policy that followed the end of World War II, dominated policy from 1945 to 1965, when it was complemented by the major financing programs. The rising costs of these interventions led in 1970 to new federal interest in reorganization, and regulatory programs followed close on its heels. Today federal health-care policy is the sum of these four strategies of intervention, each constituting a distinct political and policy "arena"; policy options are mainly variations on these established strategic and programmatic themes. (For an overview, see Table 1.)

Policy options may be viewed as rational-instrumental means to given ends, and to some extent they are. But in the real world policy choices are made and modified in multiple contexts—analytical, ethical, economic, political—that may color and distort the options' rational-instrumental appeals. In trying to shed light on the broad patterns of health-care policy, it may be useful to proceed as follows in the rest of the paper: for each of the four strategies identified here, to sketch the main "values" these contextual variables have assumed; to outline the major policy choices made and the programs that resulted; to consider the outcomes produced by these programs; to outline the central policy problems on the agenda today; and then to ponder the most prominent policy options for addressing them. This approach admittedly sacrifices depth for breadth and does not pretend to present a specialized review of the policy options, the pros and cons they entail, or the extensive literature that examines them. A broadbrush generalist treatment may, however, help to situate particular policies and possibilities in their larger settings in political time and policy space.

Subsidy

In the 1940s and 1950s policy makers debated and agreed on the proper role of the federal government in expanding the supply of health-care resources and services. The strategy authorized federal grants to sustain

Table 1   Health policy: overview of issues, options, strategies

	Subsidy (1945 –)	Financing (1965 –)	Reorganization (1970 –)	Regulation (1972 –)
Objective	Influence supply	Influence demand	Influence organization	Influence behavior
Analytic context	More is better; Supply-side strategy	Overcome financial barriers to access; Demand-side strategy	Correct faulty incentives	Assert public controls
Normative context	Attack inequities between diseases and regions	Attack inequities between classes	Meet needs more efficiently	Curb waste; Redistribute resources
Economic context	Steady growth; Fiscal conservatism; Low inflation; Low or no deficit	Strong growth; "Fiscal dividend"; Low inflation; Low or no deficit	Moderate-slow growth; High inflation; Moderate deficits	Erratic growth; Erratic inflation; High deficits
Political context	Legislative leadership; "Motherhood" issues; Breakthrough mode	Partisan, ideological, and group conflict; Breakthrough mode	"Do something": challenge but not displace status quo; Rationalizing mode	Eliminate waste; Slow red ink; Control providers; Rationalizing mode
Major theme	Build capacity	Build access	Build markets	Build controls

Major programs	NIH Hill-Burton Manpower training	Medicare Medicaid	Health Maintenance Organizations Alternative Delivery Systems in Medicaid	Professional Standards Review Organizations/ Peer Review Organizations Health Systems Agencies 1122/Certificate of Need Rate-setting/Prospective Payment System (PPS)

Major options today

Technology Assessment Control diffusion Rationing Bioethics	Medicare Retrenchment Redesign Redefinition	Experiment with Health Maintenance Organizations/Alternative Delivery Systems	Build on Peer Review organizations
Hospital capacity Tighter planning Rate setting pressure Prospective Payment System (PPS) Capacity conversion	Medicaid Transfer long-term care Federalize Expand to new groups Help states with medically indigent	Let market work Build Health Maintenance Organizations/Alternative Delivery Systems through Medicare Build Health Maintenance Organizations/Alternative Delivery Systems through Medicaid Reform health insurance market	Impose capital caps Extend and revise PPS Build new planning system
Manpower End FMGs Reduce aid Change specialities and areas Extend PPS to doctors Leave to market			

or to augment the continuing activities of, or innovation by, health-care providers, broadly defined, in particular biomedical researchers (NIH grants), hospitals (Hill-Burton), and medical personnel and the schools that trained them. It drew strength from an analytic rationale that held, in essence, that the only thing wrong with the American health-care system was that there was too little of it. A postwar venture in supply-side economics, the subsidy strategy assumed that government-supported increases in the stock of research, technology, facilities, and personnel would trickle down to underserved areas and populations and, in due course, solve problems of access without recourse to national health insurance. The rationale both reinforced and was supported by a widely shared ethical perspective. Concern ran high over, to borrow Cochrane's terms,[2] inequalities between diseases and regions. (Trickle-down was presumably to diminish inequalities between classes.) Therefore, when skeptics posed the eternal challenge to subsidy proposals—why should the federal government interpose its presence and dollars in processes that could be left to the private sector?—proponents had three replies. First, programs would address pressing, genuine national priorities—cures for dread diseases, enhanced access for the underserved, and an end to the physician shortage. Second, beneficiaries of these efforts—those who did or might suffer from cancer and the rest, the rural underserved, and those who could not get a physician when they needed one—were deserving and sympathetic. Third, neither the market nor the states and localities could be expected to do the job at the pace and on the scale desired. In short, a growing public taste for equalization generated politicization of supply-side issues (a new willingness to shift functions from the private to the public sector) and a new tolerance for centralization (general agreement that the federal government alone was up to the task). This analytical and ethical context launched the programmatic breakthroughs of the subsidy arena.[3]

Subsidy programs fit comfortably within the economic context of the 1940s and 1950s. For the most part the economy was growing steadily—between 1950 and 1960 the gross national product grew at an average annual rate of 3.2%, while the federal budget deficit averaged only about $3 billion—but even in those post-Keynesian decades fears were strong that excessive federal spending could jeopardize growth or even trigger a recession. Small, controllable project grants (NIH), formula grants (Hill-Burton), and, later, capitation grants (medical schools) promised large results without straining federal resources. (This view was correct. For example, between 1947 and 1971 the Hill-Burton program helped to build 345,000 hospital beds with an investment of $3.7 billion.[4] Medicare spent $76 billion in 1986.) These economic appeals enhanced the strategy's chief political asset, namely, that it gave policy makers eager to "do something" something to do that was neither very costly nor controversial. President Truman and the American Medical Association remained deadlocked over national health insurance, but the political properties of the subsidy programs—they engendered little partisan or ideological battling, offered potentially dramatic improvements to a population that valued them highly, had no major interest-group opponents (with the exception of the AMA in the case of federal physician training programs), and were neither technically complex nor difficult to implement—encouraged initiatives by such legislative health leaders as Representative John Fogarty (Democrat of Rhode Island) and Senator Lister Hill (Democrat of Alabama).

The dominant policy theme of the subsidy strategy, which had its heyday between 1945 and 1965, was to build capacity. Today there is general agreement that the effort succeeded, indeed in some respects too well. The federal biomedical research effort has not produced cures for the major dread diseases but it has spawned technological, pharmaceutical, and other innovations of great value. Since the 1960s, however, a growing list of caveats has counseled against expecting too much from the research effort. Technical breakthroughs have sometimes taken their place in the costly arsenal of routine practice without careful preliminary testing on cost-benefit grounds. Preoccupation with curing led to neglect of caring, perhaps a more important element of health care when one considers how many ailments have no organic source, are beyond the realm of amelioration, or get better by themselves. Costs—in money, inflated expectations, and iatrogenic illness—accompanying procedure-intensive medicine have been emphasized. Recognition of the large impact of personal preventive practices and environmental conditions on health has generated new attention to individual responsibility (in the case of prevention) and to collective societal responsibility (in the case of the environment and work place); both emphasize not medical care per se but rather the nonprovider and preinstitutional sources of health. Some have concluded that policy makers should invest fewer resources in exotic basic research and more in exhorting or inducing the population to honor Mother's insights—"Eat a good breakfast! Sleep eight hours a day! Don't drink! Don't smoke! Keep clean! And don't worry!"[5]

The shortage of hospital beds in underserved rural areas had been largely overcome by the late 1960s, and critics began to complain that the Hill-Burton program had helped to fill the nation with underoccupied, inefficient, and (in some cases) unneeded hospitals, quite without regard for the state and community planning originally envisioned. By the early 1970s the program was in political crisis: as urban and rural legislators battled over proposed changes in its allocation formula, the Nixon administration vetoed its appropriations, called for its end, and impounded its funds. In 1974 Congress ended Hill-Burton's separate legislative existence by incorporating it into the Health Planning and Resources Development Act passed that year, by which time the program had changed its priorities and was spending about 90 percent of its dollars not on new hospital construction but on modernization of old urban hospitals and construction of ambulatory facilities. Today at least 10 percent, perhaps substantially more, of the nation's bed supply is believed to be in surplus.

In the 1960s opinion polls reported the public's belief that a physician shortage was the most serious problem facing the American health-care system.[6] Federal subsidy programs helped to alleviate it so efficiently that analysts today worry about the financial implications of a serious physician surplus. In short, over the 1970s the policy question at the center of the subsidy strategy changed dramatically. Formerly, policy makers pondered the best means to expand the supply of health-care resources and services; today they seek means to constrain or to reorient that supply. In consequence, subsidy issues and options have increasingly been drawn into the regulatory arena—a major reason why regulation has remained an attractive policy option in the health field even as deregulation has come into vogue in other areas of the economy.

This policy evolution within the subsidy arena has left three general policy issues on the agenda today. Various options accompany each.

Controlling Technology

Given that medical technology is a blessing often enjoyed wastefully, what can government do to encourage production and distribution of equipment and procedures that are both more rational (better matched to the needs of the population) and more economical (more likely to yield maximum output from dollars expended)? In practice, the issue turns on devising criteria to govern the introduction, diffusion, application, and withholding of technical advances.

Option 1. Government could try to ensure that both the benefits and the costs of promising new medical techniques are carefully evaluated before they are introduced into normal practice patterns—that is, before physicians expect to use them, patients expect to have them, and payers expect to cover them. Intensive care and coronary care units, rare even in large community hospitals during the late 1950s, nearly universal by the mid-1970s, are an instructive example. Resources devoted to these units are a major element in the growth of hospital costs. Indeed, the cost of a day in an intensive care unit has been estimated to be at least three times that in a normal ward. Yet several studies comparing the progress of patients who recovered in these special units with others who convalesced in a ward or at home suggest that the benefits of intensive care and coronary care units are at best fairly small. Russell concludes that enthusiasm and faith have a sizable role in the popularity of these and other medical innovations and warns that "in the emotionally charged atmosphere of medical care, the momentum of a new technology often puts the burden of proof on those who question the evidence for it, rather than on those who propose it."[7]

One solution—perhaps the only one that can claim to be definitive—is a randomized controlled trial, whereby a procedure is simultaneously applied to and withheld from carefully matched samples of patients and the results of treatment versus nontreatment are analyzed.[8] The obstacles to extensive use of randomized controlled trials as a tool of technology assessment are well known: It is ethically troublesome to withhold from a group of potential beneficiaries the fruits of medical invention, and it is politically difficult to persuade payers to decline to pay for highly touted procedures merely because they have not been elaborately tested for several years.

These barriers to rigorous prospective assessment of procedures on the point of introduction are more understandable than the reluctance of payers and regulators to make fuller use of such "softer" retrospective assessments as cost-effectiveness analysis. Prominent as it is among payers, Medicare might be expected to lead the way in fine-tuning coverage decisions to the findings of technology assessments. Yet, as Ruby

and others point out, several factors—lack of data, lack of consideration
of cost and cost-effectiveness, unwillingness to limit coverage to specific providers and sites, and administrative problems—have kept the
program from this role.[9] Nor is Medicare's reticence merely a product of
weak political will and impoverished bureaucratic imagination. The
fundamental problem may lie in the "technology" of technology assessment itself: ". . . the methodology and procedure for determining technology 'needs' does [sic] not exist yet in generally accepted form.
Sparse data, imperfect methods of evaluating safety and efficacy, and
constantly changing technology all combine to make needs assessment
extremely difficult to perform."[10]

Option 2. The fiscal damage done by the introduction of medical
equipment and procedures of doubtful utility may be limited by constraints on the extent of their diffusion. By the same token, public and
private payers want to ensure that even cost-effective measures and
mechanisms are not distributed inefficiently among institutions and
areas. The major means by which public payers have tried to constrain
the diffusion of technologies is capital expenditure review, mainly certificate-of-need programs that require hospitals and other providers to
win the approval of a state agency before buying costly equipment. Little evidence suggests that this approach has been successful. Indeed, the
most widely cited evaluation of certificate-of-need programs found that
such savings as the programs produced by constraining the growth of
hospital beds were apparently channeled into the acquisition of new
medical equipment.[11]

The case of computerized axial tomography (CAT) scanners shows
the basic difficulties in constraining diffusion. During the middle 1970s
the peak of pressures to acquire CAT scanners coincided with the rise of
Health Systems Agencies determined to use their leverage in the certificate-of-need process to advance the cause of regional planning. A
Health Systems Agency planner in one large city described the frustra-
tions of trying to say no in that community: "Four hospitals applied for a
[certificate of need] for a new scanner. Our analysis said that only one
was justified. But the first one explained that it had been the first in the
area to purchase the original version of the scanner, which was now out-
moded. Was it going to be penalized for being farsighted? The second
noted that it was a specialty referral center for children's diseases and
could hardly keep up its quality and reputation without this equipment.

The third said it had a unique role in serving the minority population. We ended up saying yes to all three. For some reason the fourth one didn't push its application, but if it had no doubt it would've got approved too."[12]

In short, what initially appeared to Health Systems Agency staffers as questions of community need quickly transformed themselves into issues of organizational equity. Granting a new or improved CAT scanner to hospital A while denying it to hospital B would impose on B the trappings of a second-class institution and introduce (or aggravate) a status discrepancy in the hierarchy of community hospitals, which local planners and middle-range state bureaucrats were generally loath to do. Nor was there political support in the community for tough allocative rulings; on the contrary, local residents want easy access to the latest and best medical resources and rapidly lose patience with debates about optimal and efficient numbers of procedures within institutions and across regions. Looking back on their epic battles over scanners, some Health Systems Agency staffers concluded that scarce political capital had been squandered.[13] Nor is it clear that manning the ramparts against "big ticket" technologies makes sense on the merits, that is, promises large cost savings if it succeeds. Some analysts contend that the profligate repetition of small procedures such as X-rays are a much greater source of waste and their curtailment a much larger source of economies than those attending the diffusion of large, costly equipment.[14] If they are correct, policy should focus less on excessive acquisition of equipment by hospitals than on excessive utilization of procedures by physicians.

Option 3. In addition to—or perhaps instead of—trying to control the introduction and diffusion of technologies, government might work to contain the application of techniques in clinical settings. In a word, it might try to ration care. The problem has two dimensions: discouraging overutilized procedures or encouraging them to be targeted on cases in which they are likely to justify their cost, and allocating among deserving potential recipients beneficial procedures that are either too costly (artificial hearts) or too scarce (kidneys suitable for transplantation) to be made available to all who need them. In both cases there are four main rationing mechanisms: price (those who lack insurance coverage and cannot pay for procedures out-of-pocket can go without), queuing (contenders line up and are treated first-come, first-served, perhaps with some adjustment for severity of condition), chance (organs to be transplanted, for example, can be allocated by lottery), and regulation (public or private authorities can devise and apply allocation rules based on such criteria as the likelihood of survival and recovery). Among Western nations, the United States alone accepts extensive rationing by price; others prefer queuing and, in general, the stronger a nation's commitment to cost containment, the longer the queues, especially for elective surgery. Allocation of scarce benefits by lottery is endorsed by some philosophers but has so far found few enthusiasts among policy makers, who tend to prefer reasoned, rule-governed allocations in principle, but think them very difficult to devise in practice.

The policy debate on the intricacies of rationing has yet to come fully into focus for two reasons: many believe that less drastic means to contain costs—for example, technology assessment and controls on diffusion—will slow the rise of costs driven by inefficiency in the system, and such complex and costly breakthroughs as transplanted and artificial organs have generally been judged too experimental to demand authoritative policy decisions. Some analysts believe that these mitigating factors are rapidly wearing out. True cost containment will mean changes in medical practice patterns that must deprive consumers of benefits they have come to expect, and the maturing and perfecting of experimental techniques will generate demands for public rules to ensure their equitable allocation. The most important explanation for rising hospital spending, write Aaron and Schwartz, "has been technological change, which has increased the number of beneficial services." Therefore, "appreciable restraint on expenditures will be accomplished only at the price of denying medical benefits." [15]

Aaron and Schwartz's study of how hospital care is rationed in Great Britain seems to highlight three variables: the state of consumer expectations, the strength of negotiating structures in the hospital sector, and the budgetary scheme governing health-care funds. On all three counts Britain and the United States differ dramatically. The British subject is apt to wait patiently to see a physician, does not demand direct access to a specialist, and tends to accept a physician's judgment as the last word. The American "is likely to see different doctors for different problems and more frequently to regard doctors as technicians who are periodically called on to repair his physical machinery, to be dropped if they are unable to solve the current problem or to be sued if they botched the last one." The British hospital "is a quasi-feudal enterprise, ruled largely by a peerage of senior physicians . . . who usually work only at one hospital and derive most or all of their income from salary." This "select medical club" must allocate the "meager rations" the health district gives it, a process said to be "marked by compromise and trade-offs born of the recognition that each participant must spend all or most of his professional life in the company of the same colleagues." An American hospital is run by an ambiguous authority structure sharing power between administrators and medical staffs who do not leave entrepreneurial habits acquired in community practice at the hospital door. Britain finances health services by a global budget, that is, by "the simple expedient of a budget limit." The United States has established prospective per case (as in the diagnosis-related group system) or per diem limits on some hospital reimbursements, but global budgets of public funds that would put hospitals on meager rations have not been seriously entertained. Perhaps Aaron and Schwartz are right to argue that technological progress will gradually force the United States to adopt—and of course to adapt—British rationing techniques. On the other hand, a British-American comparison may be the least instructive imaginable, for both are not only off, but at opposite ends of, the curve describing normal practice among Western nations. One would expect policy lessons to emerge more readily from the experience of, say, Canada, West Germany, or France.

Option 4. The growth of meliorative technological capacity calls attention to the other side of the rationing coin, so to speak: What is appropriate policy with respect to the ardently asserted and hotly disputed "right" to refuse the application of life-prolonging medical procedures? Recently the issue has been joined at both ends of the life cycle: Do the parents of a defective newborn child have the right to decline to subject their child to medical procedures that might extend his life but could not repair severe disabilities? Does an elderly person or other adult suffering from terminal disease have the right to expect providers (presumably physicians in hospitals) to honor his "living will" declining resuscitation as death nears? Until technological progress posed these pointed ethical questions, "policy" governing such decisions tended to honor informal agreements worked out on the scene among patients, providers, parents, and clergy. Increasingly, however, the right-to-life movement has labored to persuade state legislatures that living wills usurp the divine verdict on when human life is over and to convince the federal government that to withhold treatment from a defective newborn violates a human or civil right.

In 1982, for example, the Reagan administration, disturbed by the case of an Indiana infant born with Down's Syndrome, who was allowed to die when his parents refused to authorize surgery that would easily have corrected an obstruction in his digestive tract, published rules warning hospitals that failure to give life-sustaining treatment to handicapped newborns violated section 504 of the Rehabilitation Act of 1973, which protects the civil rights of the handicapped. [16] Providers (the American Academy of Pediatrics, the American Hospital Association, and the American Medical Association among others) brought suit against the regulations, arguing that the 1973 Act had never contemplated the medical problems of handicapped newborns, and that these problems could not reasonably be handled by a civil rights approach. Despite judicial rebuffs, the administration persisted in its regulatory course, which made headlines in October 1983 as the Department of Health and Human Services tried to extract from Stony Brook University Hospital in Long Island copies of the medical records of one Baby Jane Doe, an infant born with spina bifida and several other severe problems for which corrective surgery was a controversial option the child's parents declined. The courts refused to order the hospital to surrender the records, finding that the government's creative reading of the civil rights laws was unjustified and that the parents had met the essential test in such cases—a sincere regard for the best interests of the child. Meanwhile, Congress, distressed by allegations that (as Surgeon General Everett Koop put it) handicapped infants were allowed to die in the nation's nurseries every week, and perhaps every day, amended the statutes governing child abuse and neglect in 1984 to establish new protections. The debate, which largely turns on the respective roles of abstract rights and concrete interests in ethical decisions on withholding medical technology, will doubtless grow sharper as life-sustaining procedures multiply.

Hospital Bed Supply

How should policy makers reduce the supply of beds in areas with excess capacity while taking due account of the needs of rapidly growing communities, possible economic attractions of competition among hospitals (which may require new entrants), and claims of equity and other nonpecuniary values challenged by capacity-reducing efforts? Since the early 1970s, agreement has been growing that "significant surpluses of short-term general hospital beds exist or are developing in many areas of the United States and that these are contributing significantly to rising hospital care costs." Between 1950 and 1974 the number of short-term general hospital beds nearly doubled (from 505,000 to 931,000), and the number of beds per 1,000 population climbed from 3.3 to 4.4. Using data from state Hill-Burton plans, a study group at the Institute of Medicine estimated in 1976 that at least 10 percent of the bed supply would be in surplus by 1980 and recommended that the federal government work to reduce the bed-to-population ratio from 4.4 to 4.0 per thousand within five years and "well below" that figure thereafter. [17] To date, policy makers have addressed this goal mainly by combining grass-roots planning in Health Systems Agencies (HSAs) with state-wide regulation in certificate-of-need programs. There is little evidence that the synthesis has been effective, one reason why the federal government ceased supporting HSAs and requiring state certificate-of-need laws in 1986.

The number of nonfederal hospital beds has remained fairly stable since the group issued its report. In 1975 the nation had 946,976 beds; in 1982 the number had risen to 1,015,180, falling slightly to 1,003,138 in 1985. The 4.4 beds per 1,000 population of which the group had complained in 1976 remained the same in 1982 and diminished to 4.2 in 1985. [18] Meanwhile, a national trend, sharply accentuated in the last year or two, toward fewer admissions, shorter stays, and lower hospital utilization per 1,000 population has thrust many hospitals into general fiscal stress and unprecedented competition for patients. Under the circumstances there are five major policy options.

Option I. The federal government might encourage willing states to strengthen the nexus of planning and regulation. Perhaps a firm state mandate for bed reduction and clearer instructions to local planners could produce results that are both efficient and acceptable to public opinion. The best test of this option is the evolution of the bed-reduction plan enacted by the state of Michigan in 1978. The plan, the product of a coalition of the Big Three auto companies, the United Auto Workers, and Blue Cross, who could reach consensus only on the proposition that excess beds mean excess hospital use and costs, aimed to eliminate about 10 percent of the state's bed capacity by instructing Health Systems Agencies to devise area-specific plans, meanwhile imposing a moratorium on certificate-of-need approvals in areas that failed to take action. The effort was a mixed success at best. Political bargaining with the hospitals lowered the estimated statewide surplus from 4,900 beds to 3,800 to 3,446, of which about 2,500 were located in the Detroit metropolitan region. The HSA's effort to allocate bed-reduction burdens fairly and scientifically among hospitals triggered bitter protests from small hospitals, osteopathic institutions, and, most important, from the black community, whose debate focused "not only on survival of several predominately black hospitals, but also on reemployment rights for those lower-level black hospital workers who might be displaced by hospital closures, on staff privileges for black physicians in predominately white hospitals, and, more subtly, on the tensions between the white suburban hospitals and the inner-city hospitals." Under pressure, the legislature reviewed the local plan and told the HSA to return to the drawing board. The community contemplated its revised plan and promptly went to court. Despite the stalemate, beds did close: by 1984 about 62 percent of the excess beds identified five years earlier were either gone or scheduled to close. But it is difficult to know how much this result reflected the bed-reduction effort and how much the declining fiscal condition of Detroit's center-city hospitals and voluntary negotiations over consolidations and mergers that antedated and continued alongside the legislative effort.[19] The lesson seems to be that highly democratic approaches to bed reduction—in Michigan's case, state legislation coupled with community planning—are likely to be contentious and cumbersome, proving once more that local polities value their hospitals, care little about their costs or their place in the larger system, and will fight to preserve them.

Option 2. Bed-reduction policy can be democratic without being communitarian. Instead of inviting localities to preside over the elimination of excess hospital capacity, state legislatures can establish rate-setting programs whose arcane reimbursement formulas act as an invisible hand driving marginal hospitals out of business or into mergers or consolidations. Faced, like Michigan, with serious budget pressures and extensive overbedding, New York State in 1969 adopted a prospective payment system for hospital payments to Medicaid and Blue Cross; by 1976 the system had become the most stringent in the nation.

Between 1976 and 1984 some 34 hospitals, most of them in New York City, closed their doors. The program was highly controversial. Hospitals protested that they were forced into chronic deficit, living hand-to-mouth, exhausting their endowments, and residents of poorer communities, especially in New York City, complained that their access to care and jobs was diminished. (Thorpe, however, offers evidence that as a result of the New York Prospective Hospital Reimbursement Methodology, an innovative system adopted in 1983 to govern all third-party payers, New York "successfully pursued . . . distributive goals . . . at rates of cost growth below the national average.")[20] Moreover, New York is as unique in its fashion as is Michigan. Other states with prospective hospital rate-setting programs have generally thought it prudent to stabilize and to secure the solvency of their hospitals. (New York itself has recently initiated new subsidies to hospitals to alleviate some of the burden of uncompensated care.) In Maryland and New Jersey, for example, center-city hospitals were a crucial element in the political coalition that enacted rate setting, and the program no doubt saved some of them from bankruptcy.*

Option 3. Although most states have been unwilling to use rate setting to thin hospital ranks, the federal government now has its own potent means to do so, namely, the Prospective Payment System for Medicare inpatient services adopted in 1983. A tight rein on prospective payment rates and adjustments may (as the legislative coalition that created the system believed) offer the best of both worlds: a regulatory, price-fixing scheme with strong competitive implications. Perhaps in time the incentives of the system will encourage mergers, consolidations, and takeovers, thereby eliminating much of today's surplus capacity. Possibly mindful of apocalyptic predictions directed at the hospital cost-containment plan proposed by President Carter between 1977 and 1979 (in the midst of the debate over which the Department of Health and Human Services issued controversial guidelines calling for a reduction of the nation's bed supply to four beds per thousand population), the system's supporters have said little about its capacity-reducing

---

* In New York in the late 1980s the state's political agonies over bed reduction were repaid by a bitter policy irony: the AIDs epidemic, striking with special force in New York City, imposed a heavy new demand for beds, which the frugal regulators began scrambling to add.

tendencies. A slowdown in the rate of increase in hospital spending and a decline in hospital utilization will surely be welcomed by policy makers; a rash of hospital failures and closures will probably not be.

Option 4. Policy makers might seek to make a virtue of necessity by converting excess acute-care capacity into long-term-care beds. The elderly population is growing, but nursing homes come under increasing attack as sites for geriatric care. Bruce Vladeck observed in 1980 that the numbers meshed almost exactly: by general agreement there were more than 100,000 excess hospital beds in the United States, and on any given day about 125,000 nursing home residents constituted short-stay admissions. In Vladeck's words: "It is obviously insane to build new nursing home beds when hospital beds are kept empty by the constant flow of discharges to nursing homes and only slightly less irrational to close halfway decent hospitals when fourth-rate nursing homes are entirely full. . . . The motto should be: close nursing homes not hospitals." Hospital administrators and trustees will resist this proposal, but manipulation of reimbursement—in particular higher acute-care rates for hospitals that converted excess capacity to extended-care facilities—might win support.[21]

Option 5. Do nothing. Increasingly, consumers demanding alternatives to the inconveniences and indignities of hospital care are finding a growing supply of ambulatory surgery centers and other outpatient innovations. As the interaction between supply and demand plays out, hospitals may be forced to eliminate or convert excess capacity without the assistance of explicit policy measures.

The Physician Surplus
What should policy makers do about the growing supply of physicians? That is, how can they both contain the rising costs expected to accompany those now coming on line and prevent the aggregate surplus from becoming more serious in the future? The most widely cited estimate of the magnitude of the surplus, calculated by the Graduate Medical Education National Advisory Committee (GMENAC), which reported to the Secretary of Health and Human Services in 1980, predicts a surplus of 70,000 physicians by 1990 (an increase in the number of physicians per 100,000 population from 171 in 1978 to 220) and of 145,000 (247 physicians per 100,000 population) by the year 2000.[22] Barring such approaches as that now being tried in British Columbia—refusal to

issue new insurance billing numbers to physicians judged to be in surplus[23]—five options appear to be plausible.

Option 1. At the head of most lists are constraints on the entry of graduates of foreign medical schools into practice in the United States. By GMENAC calculations, the expected arrival of 40,000 to 50,000 graduates of foreign medical schools will account for over half of the surplus expected by 1990. Another investigator argued that if the nation had ceased admitting foreign medical graduates to practice in 1986 the projected physician surplus would be eliminated by the year 2000.[24] A member of the Committee on the Size of Graduate Medical Education in New York told John K. Iglehart that such reductions are "the only palatable way to cut the number of residency training positions." Reviewing proposed legislation that would end Medicare support for foreign medical graduates seeking graduate training in the United States and would subject them to careful examination by American certifying bodies, Iglehart concluded that public and private policy is clearly headed toward sharp restrictions.[25] The potential saving in Medicare dollars and indignation over recent revelations of sales of fraudulent medical degrees have added fuel to the demographic fire. The option is not costless, however, for areas and institutions—particularly public hospitals serving poor center-city populations—that depend on foreign medical graduates. Hadley finds irony in the argument that foreign medical graduates should be limited because they provide inferior care "inasmuch as a major consequence of restricting immigration could be no care at all for people with no alternatives."[26]

Option 2. The federal government could eliminate its financial support for both medical schools and medical students. Although critics long argued that tax dollars should not be used to subsidize the entry of prosperous individuals into one of the nation's most lucrative professions, fear of the physician shortage overrode this objection during the 1960s and early 1970s. Between 1963 and 1976 five major manpower acts authorized construction funds, capitation grants, scholarships, and support for operating costs to encourage medical schools to enlarge their facilities and class size.[27] As the scope of the impending surplus became clear during the middle and late 1970s, these funds were cut considerably or made contingent on measures to promote general practice and to meet the needs of underserved areas. In the early 1980s the federal government ended all direct support for medical schools. In 1986 it reduced

Medicare payments for graduate medical education, and it has recently cut funds for student grants and loans. According to Henry A. Waxman, Democratic congressman from California, "Simply put, the federal government is no longer in the business of paying medical schools to train physicians." The government has likewise cut payments for other things the schools do, such as biomedical and behavioral research. In 1965-66 federal funds constituted over half of the revenues of the nation's medical schools; twenty years later they comprised only 25 percent of these revenues.[28] Support could be reduced further still, but this move would, needless to say, find little favor with the nation's medical schools and the universities that house them, and would do nothing to cope with the surplus already or in process of being produced.

Option 3. The federal government could try to devise both carrots and sticks to induce physicians to move from overcrowded specialties to general practice and from overdoctored affluent urban and suburban communities to inner-city and rural underserved ones. There is broad agreement that such changes are devoutly to be wished, but no practical consensus on how to accomplish them. Only 20 percent to 30 percent of American physicians are generalists (the figure depends on the definitions and measures one uses) compared to 45 percent to 80 percent in other Western nations.[29] There is limited evidence that specialists are beginning to warm to the bucolic charms of rural practice,[30] but few would assert that the "trend" is pronounced. Throughout the 1970s the federal government awarded medical school scholarships to students who agreed to serve in the National Health Service Corps after graduation, but, even before Reagan budget cuts left the corps "a moribund child,"[31] the effort was minuscule. By the late 1970s, when the nation had some 450,000 physicians, about 4,700 medical students had received National Health Service Corps scholarships. As the program began to phase out in 1982, only about 2,000 students held a scholarship or had been promised one.[32] In the late 1970s less than half (47 percent) of physicians who served in the corps remained beyond their period of obligation; by the mid-1980s only 35 percent chose to remain.[33] A reasonable inference is that general practice and underserved areas will become relatively more attractive, if ever, only when public and private payers tilt reimbursement incentives strongly in their favor. But because windfall payments to general practitioners and rural or ghetto practitioners would be costly, and a drastic suppression of payments to specialists and urban practitioners would probably be inequitable and would surely be excruciating politically, this option is likely to remain in the realm of rhetoric.

Option 4. The federal government could extend to physicians the prospective payment principle it now uses to pay for Medicare hospital services. This move would not directly reduce the physician surplus but might mitigate its costs. Current payment arrangements, which compute and pay "customary, prevailing, and reasonable" charges, have at least three disadvantages: the system contains no strong incentives to contain use and cost, does little to standardize wide and probably unjustified variations in treatment rates and costs within and between communities, and "is so complex that many physicians and most patients cannot predict what charges will be paid."[34] Various reforms are possible; each carries risks and advantages. Physicians could be paid by fee schedules or relative value scales, which reflect the payer's sense of the value of services, but physicians have "historically responded to fee controls by billing a larger number of more complex services."[35] The diagnosis-related group system now used for hospital services might be adapted to physicians. Problems arise in deciding the best object of payment—the physician as member of the medical staff, the hospital itself, or the attending physician, who would then pay other physicians who cared for the patient in question—and, whoever the payee, per-case payments might reduce physicians' incentive to treat "unprofitable" patients and ailments. Moreover, the substantial heterogeneity and variation in medical procedures could make fixed per-case payments by diagnosis-related groups inequitable, little better than "a lottery."[36] Finally, physicians could be paid by capitation—a fixed sum to cover in advance a range of services for beneficiaries. This approach virtually presupposes "a corporation that would underwrite Part A and Part B services in a state or area," but such corporations may be either unavailable or unappealing to physicians, beneficiaries, or both. Under instructions from Congress, the Department of Health and Human Services has studied these issues intensively, and they may well soon come on the agenda for serious debate.

Option 5. The federal government might elect to do nothing, allowing competition among physicians to drive costs down, either by forcing more physicians to divide the payment pie into a larger number of smaller pieces or by obliging them to protect their incomes by joining such cost-conscious plans as health maintenance organizations, or perhaps both. The hypothesis supporting this option is that the "target-income" theory, which maintains that physicians have enough discretion in defining the extent and nature of the demands they supply to multiply procedures to attain a "target income" to which they think themselves entitled, is inaccurate or, at any rate, that such behavior cannot survive competition on the scale now emerging, which is at long last creating the foundations of a well-functioning market for physician services. No one has a clue whether the target-income theory will indeed collapse as predicted by the economic optimists, but a policy of waiting to see may be an attractive last resort if consensus fails to develop around other policy options. If policy makers find merit in recent contentions that not only will there be little or no physician surplus in the closing years of this century but also that the nation might suffer a new physician shortage between 2010 and 2030, a cautious approach to further supply-suppressing measures may be highly attractive. [37]

Financing

By 1965 most policy analysts, many politicians, and much of public opinion had lost faith in trickle-down. It was increasingly clear that sizable segments of the population, especially the elderly and poor, would lack access to mainstream medical care despite substantial growth in the supply of health-care resources and facilities. The heart of the matter was financial and, having addressed inequalities by disease category and region, policy makers finally confronted the third element of Cochrane's trilogy: inequality among classes.

By the early 1960s public support was widespread for federal efforts to assist vulnerable citizens in paying their medical bills, but the moral foundations of the European and Canadian systems—that health care is a kind of civil or human right to which all citizens can claim entitlement—remained alien to American political culture. As a compromise between universalism and laissez faire and as a solution to the normative objections to "handouts" that arose whenever government proposed to pay for the housing, food, medical care, or whatever of some of the citizenry, policy makers invented what might be termed the "categorical entitlement." Medicare would cover only the elderly and would draw legitimacy from its attachment to the Social Security system, through which its hospital benefits (Part A) are financed. Thus, like Social Security, Medicare could sell itself not as a redistributive welfare program but as social insurance in which one got back what one paid in.[38] Medicaid covered a more heterogenous and less sympathetic group than the elderly, but its legitimacy would presumably be enhanced by making eligibility contingent on the close scrutiny applied to recipients of a means-tested welfare system.

Though not nearly so costly as national health insurance, these new financial commitments were very large by the standards of the day and quickly eclipsed the subsidy programs in political and budgetary prominence. The economy of the mid-1960s was in exceptional health, however. In 1960 the federal budget had a tiny ($0.3 billion) surplus, in 1965 a small ($1.6 billion) deficit; between 1960 and 1970 the gross national product grew at an annual average rate of 3.9 percent. *Mirabile dictu*, politicians feared that they could not spend the government's "fiscal dividend" fast enough to avoid "fiscal drag" on the economy, so society's capacity to afford these sizable commitments was not then in doubt. The political context similarly supported the financing strategy. Unlike subsidy programs, financing measures evoked deep partisan and ideological controversy and energetic interest-group agitation pro and con. Nonetheless, public opinion was convinced that (to blend the Democratic campaign slogans of 1964 and 1960) the federal government should "let us continue" toward a "New Frontier" of public responsibility for less advantaged citizens, and drove home its views by electing about seventy new liberal Democratic congressmen along with President Lyndon B. Johnson in 1964.[39] The categorical entitlements enacted in 1965 were a normative, economic, and political compromise that gave concrete expression to the dominant policy theme of this period: build access.

These compromises have proven remarkably stable over two troubled decades. National health insurance, widely viewed as "imminent" in the late 1960s and much of the 1970s, has faded from view. Policy makers have held sporadic debates about extending health financing benefits to new groups but, with the main exceptions of the disabled and those in need of renal dialysis (added to Medicare in 1972) and pregnant women and poor children (some of whom gained new Medicaid coverage in 1984 and 1986), neither the benefits nor the beneficiaries of the programs have changed significantly. The first major extension of benefits—to limit "catastrophic" costs of hospital services, physician care, and drugs—was enacted in 1988, more than two decades after Medicare began.

Today Medicare and Medicaid are by and large accepted as valuable programs that have brought health services to millions of citizens who would otherwise have been denied them for economic reasons. Both, however, are plainly in some degree of trouble; the central policy issue is whether their troubles constitute a "crisis" resolvable only by a major change in their character. The main challenge to Medicare lies in the interplay between demographics and costs. Table 2 outlines the growth of the program. This steady growth continues: today Medicare is the second largest federal domestic program, spending $76 billion in 1986, and is expanding fast.

Demographic trends will aggravate pressures on the program. Since 1960 the population aged 65 and over has been growing twice as fast as the younger population; the group aged 75 to 84 has grown 65 percent faster, that 85 and over 174 percent faster. In 1960, 16.7 million old people constituted 9.1 percent of the population. In 1980, 25.9 million elderly comprised 11.1 percent, and it is estimated that the figure for the year 2000 will be 36.2 million (13.2 percent), rising to 52.6 million (17.2 percent) by 2020.[40] These trends imply significantly increased demand for physicians' services and very large increases in hospital stays, nursing-home days, and expenditures.[41]

These demographic and cost pressures obviously strain Medicare's funding base. The fund ratio in the hospital insurance part of the program (funds available at the start of a year divided by disbursements during the year) declined from a peak of 70 percent in 1975 to 45 percent in 1981, which triggered predictions that the trust fund could well be exhausted between 1988 and 1996, incurring deep annual deficits thereafter.[42] A decline in the rate of inflation for health and other goods and services and diminished utilization have helped to ease the problem. The latest (1988) projections anticipate that the fund will remain in good financial health for the foreseeable future, but the demographic forecasts offer little ground for complacence.

Whereas the challenge to Medicare is to rethink how to achieve well-established and valued ends, that facing Medicaid goes to the heart of its philosophy. When the programs were enacted in 1965, policy makers pictured a general division of labor in which Medicare would assist the aged while Medicaid predominately served the younger "welfare poor." Yet largely because the joint federal-state structure of the

Table 2   Growth of Medicare, selected years

	1967	1977	1983
Number of enrollees (million)	19.5	23.8	30.0
Number of people served per 1,000 enrollees	366	570	660
Dollars reimbursed per person served	592	1,332	2,611
Dollars reimbursed per enrollee	217	759	1,724
Expenditures ($ billion)	4.5	15.6 (1975)	57.4

Source: U.S. Department of Health and Human Services, Public Health Service, *Health, United States, 1986*. DHHS Pub. No. (PHS) 87-1232, December 1986, tables 106 and 107.

program allows eligibility standards to vary with those of state welfare programs and permits benefits to differ within broad limits, Medicaid today covers fewer than half the poor. Moreover, because Medicare will pay for medical but not chronic care of the elderly, Medicaid has become the principal public source of funds for nursing-home care.

The roughly 40 percent of Medicaid dollars that goes to nursing homes meets about half of all nursing homes' expenditures, and in 1982 Medicaid spent about as much on nursing homes as on hospital care. In 1982 the aged, blind, and disabled were 28.4 percent of recipients, but used 71.9 percent of payments. Adults and children in the Aid to Families with Dependent Children program constituted 69.1 percent of recipients, but only 25.7 percent of spending.[43]

Reforming Medicare

How can the promises made under Medicare be sustained at a cost society can afford or, at any rate, tolerate? There are three broad schools of thought—retrenchers, redesigners, and redefiners—with variations on each theme.

Option 1. The federal government might try to slow the growth of its Medicare budget by reducing benefits or, more plausibly, by increasing cost sharing, in particular, higher deductibles and copayments. Although for obvious political reasons the argument is rarely stated

plainly, the assumption behind this approach is that unbridled entitlements for the aged are inefficient—they encourage the health-services
sector to consume more social resources than is desirable—and inequitable—they turn the welfare state into an elder-state without full debate
and democratic decision making as to how resources should be allocated
among claimants. In 1980 the 11 percent of the population aged 65 and
over consumed 20 percent of health-care expenditures; by 2040 the
elderly are expected to comprise 21 percent of the population and use
half its health-care dollars.[44] Granted that their needs are greater, is this
desirable or fair?

Retrenchment could take various forms, including reductions in the
number of beneficiaries (raising the initial age of eligibility or retreating
from the program's universal coverage), restrictions in the scope of services for which it will pay (which might follow implementation of findings of technology assessments, for example, or from tough reviews by
the Peer Review Organizations), cuts in payment per service (which
might reduce access by beneficiaries and strengthen providers' incentives to increase the volume of services), or—the Reagan administration's preferred approach—increased cost sharing by beneficiaries.[45]
Although Congress dismissed the administration's proposal to impose
coinsurance on the second through sixtieth days of hospital care under
the program, it agreed to increase the deductible and premium for physicians' services. According to estimates by the Congressional Budget
Office, about $7 billion of the $22 billion saved on Medicare as a result
of legislation passed in 1981 and 1982 was at the expense of the elderly,
especially the poorer elderly.[46]

Proponents of cost sharing contend that it deters excessive utilization and is in any event a painful necessity if society is to avoid the grand
collision between use and costs that appears to lie in the demographic
future. Critics counter that the elderly now have only about 45 percent of
their medical costs covered by Medicare, and conclude that if cost sharing were an effective deterrent to utilization, its effects should have been
visible by now.[47] They also exonerate demographics as the villain in the
piece. Arguing that only one-tenth of the recent growth in Medicare
physician services can be attributed to increased numbers of Medicare
beneficiaries, Marmor and Dunham remark that utilization rates rose
only "modestly" during the past decade, and infer that "medical inflation is the real culprit behind Medicare's financial instability."[48] If they

are correct, retrenchment by means of increased beneficiary cost sharing is cruel and futile.

Option 2. Some students of the program believe that it might maintain existing benefits, and even support new ones, while saving money and avoiding a resort to greater cost sharing if it were redesigned internally. One camp emphasizes redesign of its financial base. Medicare's fiscal solvency might be secured by, for example, increasing the Hospital Insurance payroll tax on employers and employees; borrowing funds from the Old Age, Survivors, and Disability trust funds; drawing more heavily on general tax revenues, especially personal and corporate income taxes; increasing taxes on such commodities as alcohol and cigarettes; introducing a value added tax; broadening the payroll tax base to include such fringe benefits as pensions, group health, and group life insurance; taxing the value of Medicare benefits for higher-income individuals; extending Social Security coverage (and financing) to all state and local employees; and taxing "medigap" policies.[49] Davis and Rowland recommend that the funding sources for Medicare Parts A and B be merged into a single trust fund, which would continue to draw payroll tax contributions and general revenues now devoted to the Health Insurance fund and Supplementary Medical Insurance expenditures, and would be complemented by a new income-related premium paid by the elderly to replace the current Supplementary Medical Insurance premium. Jack Meyer argues that parts of this proposal could be combined with "stop-loss" cost sharing scaled to ability to pay.[50] Each approach entails both advantages and liabilities for equity and efficiency, and endless permutations and combinations of elements are possible. One may probably conclude, however, that so long as the economy performs reasonably well "numerous feasible ways exist to raise substantial amounts of money" to support Medicare.[51]

A second tactic urges redesign of consumer choice in Medicare. The most widely discussed option, much favored by the Reagan administration, would give Medicare beneficiaries a voucher with which they would, after shopping around, buy health coverage from the plan of their choice, paying out of pocket for "frills" whose cost exceeds the value of the voucher. Aside from the abstract appeals of a market-oriented strategy, the approach has obvious attractions to government budget makers: it would allow them to know, indeed to set, Medicare costs in advance each year and would end haggling with providers over actual, usual, customary, prevailing, reasonable, or prospective prices of services. But these advantages should be weighed against several possible complications.

The major difficulty in a Medicare voucher system, Harold Luft points out, is adverse selection. If sicker, older, higher utilizers gravitate to higher-coverage, higher-cost plans while the healthier, younger, lower utilizers opt for less-generous plans whose premiums are closer to the value of the voucher, plan performance will "reflect not just differences in efficiency but also differences in enrollee mix." As the dynamics of self-selection favor the latter plans and damage the former, the system will "quickly fall apart." Risk adjustment by age, sex, and the like is easier said than done. There is little or no evidence that a wide range of likely competitors—independent practice associations and preferred-provider organizations, for example—will be attractive to beneficiaries or necessarily deliver high-quality, accessible care. The fine print on insurance benefits, limitations, and exclusions is difficult to communicate clearly, perhaps especially to the poor or less-educated elderly, and the larger the number of options, the more confusing the information becomes. Plans bent on building large enrollments and getting rich quickly by underserving threaten both their enrollees' health and the good name of the effort, but monitoring is "an extraordinarily complex task requiring substantial skill," which the relevant government agencies probably lack. As government fragments its bargaining leverage as a purchaser, providers may raise charges to beneficiaries, thus thwarting, at least in the short term, the cost-containment objective. Uniform national voucher levels may force residents of higher-cost regions to choose between low-option plans and high out-of-pocket costs. And, once providers find themselves fighting their economic battles not with the Health Care Financing Administration and Congress but with myriad insurers, and therefore no longer throw their political weight behind retirees and other supporters of Medicare, government budget makers may find in vouchers a good way to turn redesign into retrenchment by assuring that the growth of the value of the voucher lags behind that of the costs beneficiaries must bear out of pocket. [52]

Option 3. Medicare might be redefined to embrace new benefits. Although this may seem a utopian option in the age of Reaganomics, the inclusion of hospice benefits in Medicare in 1982 and the new program of protection against the catastrophic costs of illness enacted in 1988 show that it is not beyond the political pale.[53] One frequently mentioned candidate is preventive services, which might be defended on the same grounds as the hospice provisions, that is, as relatively low-cost services that may reduce the demand for, and the cost of, more expensive institutional care. Another possibility, of course, is long-term-care benefits, which are now largely the province of Medicaid and are best considered in the context of that program.

Reforming Medicaid

How can Medicaid be reformed to provide adequate coverage for all the non-elderly poor and medically indigent as well as or instead of the indigent elderly?

Option 1. As the figures presented earlier make clear, there are good reasons why the federal government might want to remove from Medicaid the financial burden of long-term care. The question, of course, is where else to put it. One logical course is to add a new package of long-term-care benefits to Medicare. Doing so, Anne Somers observes, would have several advantages: "It would assure neutrality of financing between acute and long-term care. It would encourage continuity of professional surveillance. It would assure access, regardless of economic status, and thus avoid promoting dependency. It would provide quality controls." As Somers also notes, however, the proposal has not been taken seriously. One reason is the cost of adding new and perhaps ambiguously defined benefits to a program already under serious budgetary stress. Another is that some analysts object to the reinforcement of the "medical model" and its acute-care paradigms that this course might entail.[54] On this view the challenge to long-term-care policy is to devise alternatives to hospitals and nursing homes—incentives for informal care-giving at home, new residential options, social health maintenance organizations, public mandating of private long-term-care benefits, new efforts by home health-care agencies—that would not easily fit into the Medicare framework and might be better promoted by demonstrations and experiments in the laboratories of the fifty states.

In 1982 the Reagan administration pushed this argument to its logical conclusion or a reductio ad absurdum (depending on one's point of view), recommending, as one version of New Federalism proposals that changed with bewildering rapidity, that Medicaid be bisected into a program covering routine care (which would become fully federal) and another for long-term care, which would become a state responsibility, supported initially by a block grant to be phased out by fiscal year 1991. The proposal found little favor. Spokesmen for the states, suspecting that they were to be stuck with the fastest-growing and least predictable and controllable costs, urged a continuing federal financial role on the grounds that "individual states with the greatest needs often do not have the resources to meet those needs."[55] City officials feared that their unusually large needs might get short shrift in the state legislature.[56] Others pointed out that the proposal would aggravate the inequities of current Medicaid arrangements: coverage and service decisions would vary among fifty states and further with their regional economies and budget cycles.

The limitations of fully federal and fully state-run approaches suggest that a synthesis combining federal fiscal capacity with state innovation in service delivery would be preferable. Somers recommends that amendments eliminate from Medicare the prohibition against chronic care and that a defined set of institutional and home-based long-term-care benefits be added. Prospective payments to providers and some cost sharing by beneficiaries would help hold down costs. Simultaneously, a federal-state-local program to coordinate long-term-care services would be created, its purpose being "to provide comprehensive assessment, appropriate placement, and cost-effective case management of individual long-term patients under the general supervision of a responsible primary physician or group," or some other suitable mechanism.[57] Other analysts would fashion new private solutions, for example, reverse equity mortgages in which older homeowners receive monthly payments from financial institutions in exchange for all or a portion of the equity in their homes. This approach, like long-term-care insurance and other market-oriented answers, does little to address the needs of the less affluent, which would surely require a sizable commitment of new public funds.

Option 2. The federal government might "federalize" Medicaid, that is, establish a uniform set of benefits and eligibility standards the states would be obliged to honor and, because state fiscal capacities differ, assume full financing of the program. The normative argument for this option is straightforward: how can it be right that a sick American citizen who happens to reside in Mississippi should find it harder to get public assistance and should receive a smaller range of medical services once he gets it than a citizen who happens to live in New York? Critics have railed against these "disparities and inequities" for years with little result. One reason is that federalizing Medicaid raises the same policy issues as do proposals to reform welfare by such means as a family-assistance plan, guaranteed annual income, or negative income tax, and faces the same obstacles. State fiscal capacities and ideological preferences on the proper role of welfare (including Medicaid) in American society differ. Uniform benefit and eligibility standards must compromise among existing state practices, and concrete proposals invariably offer benefits too high for conservatives, too low for liberals (including states with very generous benefits) and come accompanied by eligibility standards too lax for the former, too strict for the latter. In a European system these disagreements would be resolved within the ruling party or coalition; in the American system they cut across party lines and no leadership structures are strong enough to break the deadlock. In the United States, too, a problem of political strategy has compounded the policy confusion. By and large those most favorable to federalizing Medicaid are also those most committed to comprehensive national health insurance and have feared that a better Medicaid program would remove a major argument for broader reform.

Option 3. The federal government could incrementally expand the system of categorical entitlements by creating new or expanded benefits for existing eligibles, authorizing or easing eligibility for new groups, or both. As to new benefits, consider a federal study of the health of minority groups, which recently reported a "persistent, distressing disparity" in death rates by race in the United States, including a black infant mortality rate twice that of whites, and recommended that Medicaid benefits for prenatal care be expanded.[58] The recommendation is at once unexceptionable and troubling. Pondering a recent epidemiologic study of racial and socioeconomic differences in child mortality in Boston, Robert J. Haggerty concluded that perhaps expanded personal health services should take a back seat to (for example) gun control, enforcement of housing standards, requirements for smoke detectors, a higher drinking age, and stronger efforts to equalize incomes.[59] Nor is this a dilemma brought on solely by the penurious policies of the Reagan administration. Personal health services are fully capable of consuming every discretionary dollar available to the American welfare state, and services that appear to be unquestionably deserving of expansion within the context of Medicaid become problematic when viewed as part of the big picture.

Because fewer than half the poor qualify for Medicaid (in good part because more than half the states set income eligibility standards below $5,000 for a family of four), many new groups might be included in the program—for instance, the two-parent poor and the medically indigent in states that do not cover them, unemployed people who lose their health benefits when (or soon after) they lose their jobs, the 10 percent to 15 percent of the population with no health insurance at all, and those who incur the costs of catastrophic illness. Each group constitutes a moral and political universe of its own (that, indeed, is part of the problem) and each has been the subject of inconclusive policy debates. The debates have been inconclusive for several reasons, including disagreement about the severity of the problem (how many unemployed workers shift to health coverage under a spouse's policy?) and about the best mechanism for dealing with it (how far could the government go toward solving the problem of the uninsured by mandating coverage by private employers?), and anxiety over the effects of piecemeal reform on a comprehensive solution (a source of concern when national health insurance was considered a live option) and over the effect of proposed solutions on the federal budget deficit. Today these groups are increasingly lumped together under the headings "medically indigent" and "uninsured," and their problems are consigned by the Reagan administration (by choice) and by liberals (by necessity) to the states.

Option 4. The federal government could defer to or encourage state efforts to address the problem of indigent care. Several strategies are available.[60] First, states and their local communities can try to develop new health insurance offerings that small businesses might buy for their otherwise uncovered workers. With the assistance of a Robert Wood Johnson Foundation program for the medically uninsured, fifteen state and local sites are now experimenting with variations on this and similar themes. Although this strategy may identify or create new harmonies of interest between some insurers and employers, many others will probably continue to decline to sell or buy. Therefore, second, states may elect to mandate that all but the smallest firms offer health insurance to their workers. Hawaii initiated this approach in 1974 and in April 1988 Massachusetts adopted it with great fanfare. Alaska, Maine, and Rhode Island require that employers offer their workers coverage for catastrophic illness. Mandating, however, leaves unassisted people who have neither a job nor health insurance, which (third) argues that states should expand Medicaid eligibility and services, as Michigan, Wisconsin, South Carolina, and several other states have done. But even an enlarged Medicaid program is unlikely to cover all the poor, so, fourth, states may subsidize hospitals that deliver burdensome amounts of uncompensated care by redistributing the proceeds of an assessment on the revenues of all hospitals (Florida, West Virginia, South Carolina), incorporating allowances in hospital rate-setting programs (New York, New Jersey, Maryland), or in other ways. In the absence of universal, uniform benefits adopted by the central government, no single solution will suffice. Each state will be obliged to mix and match these fourfold elements into a strategy that meets its particular needs and preferences.

Those distressed by the unwillingness of the federal government to take on the problem may applaud the states' energy and ingenuity; the "laboratory" of the American federal system appears to be alive and well. Those troubled by the wide variety of approaches under discussion and trial may complain that the essence of equity—the citizen's "right" to standard benefits under uniform eligibility criteria—is fading further from view.

Reorganization

By 1970 it had become clear that the federal commitment both to augment the supply of health-care resources and services and to finance the demand of a part of the population for those resources and services was a costly proposition. The array of programs, each defended by political participants eager to protect their preserve, seemed increasingly to mire the policy process in (to borrow a term from Samuel H. Beer) "pluralistic stagnation." As the 1970s proceeded, debate centered less on potential new additions to the federal agenda (breakthroughs), more on how to improve the workings of what was already on it, that is, "rationalizing" policies.

Targets for rationalization were numerous, but policy analysts focused in particular on the effects of the system by which the growing corps of providers was paid in the financing programs—retrospective calculation of the costs or charges of individual services and reimbursement of those judged to be "reasonable." Critics asserted that these arrangements offered a blank check to providers, whose incomes varied directly with the volume of services they rendered and who faced no incentives to practice in a cost-conscious fashion. This economic logic carried disturbing normative implications. The federal government probably could not afford indefinitely to honor the entitlements it had confidently conferred on the elderly and poor in 1965. Some analysts, however, urged a solution that seemed almost intuitively obvious. If the system's incentives were changed to encourage greater efficiency by providers, everyone could enjoy every service to which he laid legitimate claim. Thus began in earnest the effort to reinterpret equity in the light of efficiency.

The economic context of the early 1970s supported the quest for savings by corrected incentives instead of the "dead hand" of public regulation. Inflation was worrisome (enough so to drive the Nixon administration to wage and price controls in 1971) but growth was respectable (the gross national product increased by an annual average of 2.9 percent over the decade) and the federal budget was under control (in 1970 the deficit was only $2.8 billion). Thus, policy makers sought systemwide savings, not sharp sudden cuts in public spending. The political context also favored saving by incentives, markets, and competition. There was diffuse concern about the "crisis" of rising health-care costs but no consensus for basic changes imposed by government. Under the circumstances, policy makers welcomed proposals that embodied "correct incentives" in a concrete organizational framework—what came to be called "alternative delivery systems" that would challenge and change the existing system without displacing it. The dominant theme of the early 1970s, revived a decade later, was building markets.

Though policy makers in 1970 seemed to view market building as a relatively painless, low-conflict endeavor, they had poor grounds for this expectation. In the Medicare law in 1965 and again in the statute establishing the Regional Medical Programs in 1966, the federal government assured the medical profession that it would stay out of the delivery and organization of health care; the federal infatuation with reorganization was a major political departure. To be sure, on occasion the federal government had developed new organizations to bring care to special populations—for instance, the health system run by the Veterans Administration, the neighborhood health centers launched by the Office of Economic Opportunity and the Model Cities program, and (in

1972) the National Health Service Corps to bring physicians to under-served areas. The reorganization effort contemplated in the early 1970s, however, broke with this pattern, too, for its aim was to trigger broad systemwide reforms that would save money for society as a whole without sacrificing access or quality. Established providers warned that government ventures into this uncharted terrain could upset their settled expectations and those of consumers, and decried the unfairness of federal financial and other support for competitive systems. Policy makers replied that they intended not to displace the status quo, but merely to subject it to the bracing challenge of competition and market discipline—precisely what was needed, for the status quo was increasingly viewed as part of the problem, not the solution.

The main programmatic product of this enthusiasm for reorganization was federal legislation to promote health maintenance organizations. Between 1970 and 1972 Congress tried, with limited success, to agree on ways to ease enrollment of Medicare beneficiaries in HMOs. In 1973 new legislation authorized federal grants, loans, and other advantages to help them to take root across the nation. For various reasons, the federal HMO development effort was slow to take off, controversial, and much amended.[61] Upon entering office the Reagan administration concluded that direct federal aid to them was unnecessary and began phasing it out.

Today there is much uncertainty about both the accomplishments and the potential of HMOs and other variants such as independent practice associations and preferred-provider organizations (PPOs) that collectively comprise alternative delivery systems and stand at the center of the so-called competitive strategy. Although there is little firm evidence on the cost-containment accomplishments of PPOs, their growth has been explosive. At the end of 1984 there were 141 of them, 106 in operation, 35 under development. They were located in 29 states, the District of Columbia, and Puerto Rico; 52 were located in California.[62] By mid-1988 there were 646 PPOs, 608 in operation, 38 in development. They were in 43 states; 110 were located in California.[63]

Evidence on the progress and effects of HMOs is more abundant but far from definitive.[64] Their growth has accelerated in the late 1980s but is still very limited in view of the high expectations of their enthusiasts. In the early 1970s, when the federal government began promoting HMOs, there were 100 of them, enrolling about 2 percent of the population.

After more than a decade of hope and hype, there were, at the end of 1983, 290 plans with almost 14 million members—about 6 percent of the population. By September 30, 1987, the numbers had roughly doubled: 662 HMOs were serving about 29 million members—about 12 percent of the population. Membership is highly concentrated in plans and regions, however. Fifty-two percent of enrollees were in one of the 62 plans with 100,000 or more members; about one-third of that 52 percent belonged to one of the 12 Kaiser plans, 7 of which exceed 100,000 members. Eleven states have 54 percent of the plans and 65 percent of the nation's HMO enrollment. California has about 8 percent of the plans and 25 percent of the membership. Only 21 states and the District of Columbia have an HMO with more than 100,000 members.[65]

Although there is a respectable record that HMOs—at any rate sizable and mature-group or staff-model ones—register impressive internal efficiencies, little evidence suggests that their presence, even in communities in which they have won substantial penetration, has produced savings in the larger system. Examining competitive dynamics in Hawaii, Rochester, and Minneapolis-Saint Paul (the Twin Cities), Harold Luft reports that "the absence of a cost-containment effect" or that a cost-containing response will be "slow and uncertain." In a study of the Twin Cities, Johnson and Aquilina report "no clear evidence of communitywide utilization-reducing effects directly attributable to the 'competitive effect' " of health maintenance organizations; that is, their growth through 1981 "had not significantly affected overall hospital costs, revenues, or profits." Studying the Twin Cities between 1979 and 1981, Feldman concluded that HMOs' sizable growth and competition did not restrain hospital expenditures per admission as competition advocates expected, and argued that if competition is to work it must go well beyond HMOs. Assessing the impact of competition in a sample of Standard Metropolitan Statistical Areas, Merrill and McLaughlin showed that growth of HMOs led to a lower level of hospital admissions, but also to a higher level of hospital expenses per capita (not merely per case), and could find no influence on the rate of growth of hospital expenses per capita or per patient day. Their conclusion: "The extent of HMO penetration in a community does not appear to have had any significant spillover effect on reducing overall hospital costs."[66]

Though hardly a policy and perhaps not even a strategy, competition is a fact of life today, but its causes and consequences are controversial and little understood. Competition—meaning here efforts by physicians, hospitals, and insurers to attract consumers by appeals to price as well as other amenities—is a result of the convergence of several distinct though related developments peaking in the mid-1980s. Public and official anxiety over devoting more than 10 percent of gross national product to health, over an annual national health budget threatening to hit $1 trillion in the early 1990s, and over the supposedly impending depletion of the Medicare hospital insurance trust fund created a general sense that deep-reaching reforms were desirable. Accumulating data depicting the wide variation in the rates and costs of treatment within and between areas—variations that have no evident medical justification—challenged the traditional view that every medical decision reflects pristine scientific professionalism and suggested instead that a sizable amount of the care rendered and the cost paid is "arbitrary and capricious." Further data compiled, analyzed, and publicized by professional standards review organizations, rate-setting bodies, health-systems agencies, and private data firms systematically compared peer groups of physicians and hospitals, pinpointing who performed and charged more, who less. Increasing availability of these data in the computers of large purchasers, especially business firms, gave them confidence that they could accurately identify "preferred providers" and emboldened them to contract accordingly. The diffusion of coalitions and communication networks such as the Washington Business Group on Health spread the word on these and other cost-containment techniques within the business community. The conviction that economic discipline presupposes organizational discipline fueled enthusiasm for reorganization and gave rise to a managerial imperative that may be as important in the 1980s and 1990s as was the technological imperative in the 1970s and the access imperative in the 1960s. Finally—largely as an unintended consequence of federal subsidy programs—the growing surplus of hospital beds and physicians deprived these providers of the power and in many cases the will to resist the new purchaser pressures. These trends have generated, helter-skelter, a host of competitive projects that fall along a continuum running from efforts to build such comprehensive and integrated organizations as health maintenance organizations; to agreements to accept utilization review and discounted fees by lists of physicians in independent practice associations and preferred-provider organizations; to entrepreneurial schemes by individual hospitals to secure patient "markets" by means of advertising, speciali-zation, diversification of investments, and horizontal or vertical integra-tion with corporate chains; to efforts by individual corporations to self-insure, that is, offer their own insurance plans to their employees and eliminate the Blue Cross or commercial middlemen. It is too soon to tell which, if any, of these highly heterogeneous competitive endeavors will last, which will contain costs, and which, if any, will be judged socially desirable. The role that public policy can play in these compli-cated happenings is also problematic.

Alternative Delivery Systems

Given the equivocal evidence on systemwide savings by such compara-tively well-analyzed organizations as HMOs, and given that alternative delivery systems embrace organizations and arrangements very differ-ent from them and little understood, should the federal government embrace such systems as a policy strategy and work to promote them?

Option 1. Some propose that the federal government assist in the design and funding of carefully drawn experiments, demonstrations, and evaluations that rigorously assess the cost-saving effect of HMOs and other alternative delivery systems in local communities. Others argue that competition has been working for a long enough time and on a wide enough scale in Hawaii, the San Francisco Bay region, and the Twin Cities to support conclusions about the strategy and that it has been found wanting, at least for purposes of cost containment in the larger system. As for other alternative delivery systems, this school would contend that an experimental regimen could not possibly tell federal pol-icy makers all they need to know to act sensibly before the pressures to act precipitously overwhelm them.

Option 2. The federal government could admit that it has at hand no acceptable strategy to promote alternative delivery systems directly and could defer to the market dynamics now on display in the private sector. On this view the federal determination to play the prudent purchaser in prospective payment systems advances the cause of efficiency and com-petition as much as reasonably can be done. Having unintendedly pro-moted competition by helping to create a surplus of physicians and hospital beds, it should now allow alternative delivery systems to develop however the market ordains.

If the federal government wants directly to encourage alternative delivery systems in the short term, how can it best do so when its own financial leverage is largely limited to Medicare and Medicaid?

Option 1. The federal government can try to enlarge the enrollments and coffers of health maintenance organizations by easing the way for Medicare beneficiaries to enroll in them. Today only about 3.5 percent of this group belongs to one, in part the legacy of continuing conflict between payment norms in HMOs—prospective premiums per enrollee to cover a comprehensive range of services—and in Medicare—retrospective reimbursement for allowable costs. After more than a decade of debate and lobbying, the HMOs in 1982 finally won provisions in the Tax Equity and Fiscal Responsibility Act (TEFRA) that allow them to receive prospectively premiums equal to 95 percent of the amount Medicare would expect to spend per enrollee in the traditional system. "Profits" (that is, the difference between the 95 percent payment and what it costs the organization to serve the beneficiary) must be used to reduce premiums or enlarge benefits; any losses are absorbed by the HMO. Some observers predict that these amendments will trigger a mass migration of the elderly to HMOs, but unforeseen problems have arisen. Fearing that conversions of beneficiaries already enrolled under the old "cost" contracts could cost the government $200 million to $300 million in the first year of the program, the lawmakers wrote into TEFRA a "two-for-one" rule: HMOs caring for the elderly under cost contracts must enroll two new members under the "risk" arrangements before converting existing members to the option. Thus the Kaiser plans in California each would be obliged to enroll 260,000 new Medicare members before they could offer their present 130,000 members the advantages of the new arrangements, which is not only inequitable but also an inducement to existing members to find a new plan. The provision poses no major problem for HMOs with few Medicare enrollees under a cost contract but even these fear "diddling" with rates when the Health Care Financing Administration begins wondering why it should pay 95 percent of conventional costs to plans that can deliver care for 85 percent or less.[67] Short-term budget savings and long-term promotion of HMOs may conflict. Some analysts believe that the trade-off could be largely dispelled if the government adopted a Medicare voucher system in which HMOs could directly display their competitive appeals, but this approach has problems of its own, discussed earlier.

Option 2. The federal government can continue to give the states leeway to try alternative delivery systems in Medicaid. Since the 1970s that program has been subjected to cross-pressures that create much policy confusion. Its rising costs mean that it cannot be eliminated. Its domination by long-term care means that its original philosophy— assuring access to mainstream care for the welfare poor and the medically indigent—cannot be preserved, but recurrent scandals surrounding Medicaid mills and client abuse mean that it must be reformed. In the Omnibus Budget Reconciliation Act of 1981 Congress in essence threw up its hands, imposing modest funding cuts while extensively enlarging the states' discretion to experiment with alternative delivery systems in Medicaid.

Today "managed care" is a watchword of Medicaid policy. The approach usually entails some combination of such elements as "gatekeeping" roles for generalist physicians, on whose approval a referral to a specialist is contingent; capitation payments to organized plans (including HMOs) awarded Medicaid contracts by competitive bid; "lock-ins" of clients to one of a defined universe of service providers instead of the freedom of choice once thought to be inseparable from "mainstream" care; requirements of prior authorization by primary-care physicians before a patient is admitted to a hospital; and increased use of cost sharing to deter excessive use.[68] It is, of course, too soon to draw conclusions about the costs and benefits of these arrangements, but in time they are likely to be a rich source of instruction on the workings of alternative delivery systems.

Critics argue that these special arrangements for the Medicaid population amount to an unrepentant retreat from the equal access to mainstream care toward which the federal government should be working. Some defenders—spokesmen for the Reagan administration, in particular—are content to declare that equality has had too much attention as a policy objective; the United States has a two-tiered system, and will continue to have one as a matter of economic necessity, but adequate care is achievable within that constraint. Others contend that sensible policy demands a more sophisticated explication of the question, "Equal access to what?" Surveying the system's chronic inability to reconcile its allegiance to egalitarianism in the allocation of care with libertarianism in the conditions of its production, Uwe Reinhardt concludes that the notion of equal access most consistent with American social values "implies that the probability of surviving a medical condition after medical treatment, and the degree of recovery, be independent of the patient's socioeconomic and insurance status but that the amenities accompanying the delivery of care and the degree of freedom of choice among providers may vary systematically by socioeconomic class.[69] One might reply that the correlates of health status outcomes are usually the last thing on the minds of those designing alternative delivery systems for state Medicaid populations, and that it can be difficult to draw the line between amenities and the qualitative dimensions of care (in which category, for instance, is a reasonably leisurely chat with the physician taking a medical history?), but Reinhardt's proposition nicely formulates an issue that will be high on the policy agenda for a long time.

Pro-competitive Reforms
If the federal government decides that it wants to advance the cause of alternative delivery systems and hopes to do so by quicker and more authoritative means than those available to it in Medicare and Medicaid, how might it reform the national health insurance market (and perhaps other aspects of the system) to achieve this end?

Option 1. For more than a decade policy makers have discussed various legislative measures that might create new opportunities for consumer choice in the context of "correct" incentives in the health insurance market. The usual list includes: a federal requirement that employers who provide health insurance for their workers offer a choice of several different plans; that employers make equal financial contributions to each plan, obliging employees who prefer "less efficient" alternatives to pay a portion of the extra cost out of pocket; that a dollar cap be placed on the value of health insurance premiums paid by employers on behalf of workers that is excluded from the taxable income of the latter; and perhaps a tax or cash rebate to employees who sign on with more efficient plans. These options have been opposed by business, labor, hospitals, physicians, insurers, the elderly, and health maintenance organizations, and they have conceptual as well as political problems. A central one is the adverse selection likely to set in when younger, healthier, low-utilizing subscribers are drawn to cheaper plans with narrower benefits and higher cost sharing while the older, sicker, high-users move into more generous plans (such as HMOs) with broader benefits and less cost sharing but higher premiums. To offset this danger the government could impose restrictions and uniform standards on

benefit schedules, recruitment practices, and premium-setting methods
for all plans, as Alain Enthoven has proposed.[70] This approach is too
regulatory and too redolent of national health insurance to find favor
among the Reaganites, however.

The administration has pushed hard for one element of the pro-competitive package, the cap on the tax exclusion. Originally it would have
treated as taxable income all employer-paid health insurance premiums
above $70 per month for individuals and $175 per month for families,
which would have affected about 30 percent of workers and raised about
$30 billion over four years. In the heat of skirmishing over tax reform in
the spring of 1985 the executive branch recommended instead a tax on
the first $25 of employer-paid health insurance for all workers who
receive it.

The cap has found favor among economists for reasons of equity—
the exclusion discriminates against citizens who do not have work-
related health insurance, and is regressive because its value rises with
income—and of efficiency—the exclusion encourages workers to buy
excessive health insurance, and its reform could help reduce the deficit.
The proposal has been sharply attacked, however, by an unusual coalition of the left, arguing that the cap imposes a new tax on working and
middle-class Americans, and the right, contending that by weakening
the market for private health insurance and encouraging shallower coverage it would drive the nation down the road to national health insurance. In deliberating on the tax reforms enacted in 1986, Congress
debated the proposed cap at some length, but neither the House nor the
Senate came close to passing it. Indeed, today this last residuum of federal pro-competitive legislation appears to be about as imminent as
national health insurance.

Regulation

Regulation is a strategy with large policy appeals and equally large
political liabilities. To policy makers hoping quickly to contain costs
that keep rising despite their best pro-competitive efforts, regulatory
controls seem to go to the heart of things. But government "interference" in private-sector processes is much resented by those subjected to
it, and a huge analytical literature warns that nothing works out as antic-
ipated in the regulatory world.

By the early 1970s and increasingly over the decade analysts concluded that the many well-known market imperfections in the health-care system put major obstacles before competitive solutions, at least any with a shred of political plausibility. Moreover, mounting evidence on variations in the rates and costs of treatment suggested that providers were sometimes indifferent to or too little concerned about the cost of care. The implication was that government had little choice but to inter-vene directly to constrain (though not of course to dictate or determine) the decisions of providers about utilization, quality, pricing, and con-struction and expansion of facilities.

The normative inference was unsettling: each citizen might hope to enjoy all the care he needed at a price society could afford only if the system as a whole were changed in important respects, and not by the invisible hand of correct incentives but rather by governmental design. The price of equity came to be viewed as a redistribution of resources whose theme was the deliberate elimination of waste, certainly among providers, perhaps among consumers too. Providers countered with their own normative critique: regulation takes too little account of regional, state, and local variations and needs; inflicts the heavy hand of bureaucracy on delicate economic mechanisms; and entails a host of inequities, inefficiencies, and perversities. Policy makers replied in effect that society could not afford *not* to regulate; someone had to "do something" and no one knew what else to do.

In the early and middle 1970s the economic context—high anxiety about inflation but little concern about the federal budget deficit—sup-ported only mild and tentative regulatory experiments. In the early 1980s, however, health costs rising at two or three times the rate of gen-eral prices combined with huge budget deficits to generate a new climate that supported the quest for stronger regulatory tools even if these entailed significant changes in reimbursement and delivery patterns. The political context was similarly favorable. Politicians had patiently experimented with health maintenance organizations, had waited in vain for the Reagan administration to offer comprehensive pro-competi-tive legislation, had monitored the meager accomplishments of the weak, decentralized regulatory programs of the 1970s, had witnessed the hospital industry's unsuccessful voluntary effort to slow the growth of costs, had studied piles of evidence on waste and overuse in the sys-tem, and now were increasingly resolved that the federal government would use its potential as a prudent purchaser to curb its own costs and in the process pressure the larger system to mend its ways. The dominant policy theme by the early 1980s, in short, was building controls.

The programmatic outputs of this regulatory evolution have centered on four generic types of control: utilization review, planning, capital expenditure review, and rate setting. Utilization review (which many hospitals had adopted voluntarily before Medicare and Medicaid required it in the late 1960s) gained a cost-containment emphasis, albeit an ambiguous one, with the enactment of legislation in 1972 establishing Professional Standards Review Organizations; in 1982 these were transformed into new, supposedly stronger Peer Review Organizations. In 1974 the Health Planning and Resources Development Act built Health Systems Agencies (HSAs) on the foundations of the effete Comprehensive Health Planning Agencies created in 1966. The same legislation also required that all states adopt certificate-of-need programs to regulate capital expenditures; at that time about half the states already had such laws. In 1972 the federal government extended financial support and technical assistance to state programs that set hospital rates prospectively, and late in the 1970s it waived Medicare and Medicaid payment rules for some rate-setting states. In 1983 it adopted its own prospective payment system for inpatient services in Medicare, based on the diagnosis-related groups that had been put most fully into practice in New Jersey's rate-setting program.

Today there is considerable agreement that rate setting by means of prospective payment seems to "work" (that is, helps contain costs)[71] but that utilization review, planning, and capital expenditure review do not—at least on the evidence of the quantitative evaluations of the programs listed above. Rate setting has spread at the state level and to the federal level. Despite its achievements in reducing the rate of growth of spending for inpatient services, it is far from clear that rate setting is an adequate method of cost-containment, however. As the 1980s end, "squeezing the balloon" is an increasingly common image. Prospective payment systems hold the line on inpatient use and revenues, but outpatient services and spending rise dramatically. Aggressive employers strike favorable deals with hospitals and insurers, who recoup by increasing charges to buyers with less bargaining acumen or leverage. Costs for some routine procedures level off; costs for mental health services skyrocket. In the 1990s policy makers are likely to debate hitherto heretical means of slowing the flow of dollars into the system by imposing controls on both use and price for the full range of payers, providers, and consumers. Budgetary regulation may well take forms more stringent than those of the 1970s and 1980s, and will probably supplant behavioral regulation (detailed monitoring of utilization and capital expenditures) as the cost-containment strategy of choice.[72]

Meanwhile, it is unclear whether the other approaches have failed to contain costs because they are inherently flawed or because the programs embodying them were poorly designed.[73] Many analysts have argued the former, but policy makers have generally acted as if they believed the latter. Instead of eliminating the professional standards review approach, as the Reagan administration recommended, Congress chose to fashion peer review organizations. Until 1986 Congress likewise declined to kill the health planning program. Although many HSAs have closed their doors, local cost-containment coalitions have sprung up across the nation. Whereas the HSAs were concerned above all with establishing countervailing power between providers and consumers, the local community coalitions give new voice to the *payers,* a development that could change the politics of cost-containment if purchasers should one day overcome their customary commitment to the maintenance and growth of the hospitals on whose boards they sit and their usual aversion to adversarial relations with providers. The nature of certificate-of-need programs varies among the states, as it always has. In some states capital expenditure regulation is in retreat, but in others—Michigan and New York, for example—it has led to a debate on the wisdom of legislatively imposed ceilings on capital expenditures, which would force decisions to be based not on the elastic criterion of community "need" but rather on the more tangible and constraining criterion of affordability. In short, despite the antiregulatory rhetoric of the Reagan administration, the regulatory strategy is alive and well. This is all the more the case because (as argued above) many current issues related to subsidies and financing have assumed a regulatory complexion.

Unfortunately, the policy significance of this regulatory evolution has been obscured by the preoccupation of some analysts with market-oriented consequences, that is, with the effectiveness of regulation as a means of containing undesired market effects or of mimicking the desirable effects markets would produce if they were working well. The larger consideration is that accessible care of acceptable quality can be harmonized with the containment of costs in any system with extensive third-party payment only if payers (public, private, or both) build stable negotiating structures with providers. This view, obvious to Europeans, comes hard to Americans, who may believe (on the left) that governmental purposes should remain untainted by private interests or (on the right) that government interference inevitably leads either to the capture of the regulatory entity or to the destruction of the virtues of the marketplace. American providers have shared this antipathy to negotiation, understanding that it would mean that government involvement is here to stay, and that give-and-take with payers would replace lofty appeals to professional privilege. Before the enactment of Medicare American providers had no need or occasion to bargain with the federal government; after its passage, the problem was "solved" by the compromise accepting retrospective cost and charge-based reimbursement. In the 1970s, however, policy makers invented regulatory programs that began to draw providers into loosely structured dialogues about proper standards and norms for the use of hospital care; logical relations between needs and resources in communities, regions, and states; the community's need for new or renovated facilities and equipment of different types; and the reasonableness of the relations among hospital costs, services, and prices. In the 1980s public and private payers have increasingly found confidence and voice and in their "corporate" capacity as payers have insisted that providers engage in more tightly structured negotiations. The regulatory programs have advanced this trend; indeed, regulation is one name under which structured negotiations are evolving; competition is another.

Building Regulatory Capacity
How can government use regulatory programs both as constraints on providers and as structures for negotiation on how society can contain increases in the cost of care without unacceptable sacrifices in access and quality?

Option 1. The federal government could rely more heavily on utilization review, which taps the legitimacy and leverage of physicians' self-regulation to persuade "high rollers" to practice a more frugal style of medicine. The professional standards review organizations, which were not notably effective in containing costs, suffered several liabilities. The federal government did not clarify the relative emphasis they were to put on cost versus quality considerations. The organization-building process itself, which included informing local physicians, recruiting staff, establishing formal procedures, gathering and analyzing data, debating about norms, standards, and criteria for review, and inducing hospitals to cooperate, took time and required extensive compromise. The commitment to localism in some 200 such organizations assured highly heterogeneous outcomes. The federal decision to fund the plans by grants virtually assured that weaker sisters would be "carried," for the alternative was to start all over again building a new organization. The new peer review organizations may learn from the unhappy lessons of their predecessors. The federal government has made it plain that they must demonstrate cost savings. They can build on the organizational foundations, skills, personnel, and communications networks of the professional standards review organizations. There is one peer review organization per state, not four times that number in diverse localities. And they are funded by contracts that, the government has warned, will be withdrawn and awarded elsewhere if one fails to deliver. Some critics remain convinced that physician self-discipline in economic matters will always be lax and half-hearted at best. Other observers expect few savings from peer review organizations but believe that they can fulfill two other important functions: educating physicians about variations in practice patterns and charges among their peers and monitoring the quality of care.

Option 2. The federal government could legislate an annual dollar ceiling on capital expenditures by the states (as the Carter cost-containment plan of 1977 proposed to do) or require that each state adopt and enforce a ceiling of its own. The demand of local communities and their institutions for new construction, expansion, renovation, and acquisition and upgrading of medical equipment is virtually unlimited, and so are the costs of indulging these expansionist tastes. Certificate-of-need reviews, which examine each proposal on its individual merits, concentrating attention on whether it addresses a community "need," seldom issue denials and at best postpone the costs of large capital commitments by delaying approvals. Moreover, some critics argue that certificate-of-need reviews should not ask whether the community "needs" one or another improvement (of course it does) but rather whether, given its larger priorities and limited resources, it can afford them. In short, certificate-of-need review should be redesigned to address "relative" not "absolute" need, and perhaps the only way to force policy makers and institutions to change the nature of reviews is to limit available resources by some type of dollar cap.

Some states—Michigan and New York, for example—have imposed temporary moratoria on new certificate-of-need approvals while debating capital caps, but none has yet adopted one, presumably from fear that public opinion will not accept the austerity or the blood-letting among institutions a cap might entail. Yet it is hard to see how capital expansion and its attendant increases in operating costs and utilization can be slowed without ceilings on the number of dollars allowed to flow into the system.

Option 3. The federal government could concentrate its regulatory energies on refining and extending the prospective payment approach. Instead of relying on physicians to curb their own utilization or on states to deny their own communities' preferences for modern, growing hospitals, the federal government might use its leverage as a major purchaser to slow the flow of dollars into the system. The shift from retrospective to prospective payment in Medicare is widely viewed as the most important health-policy decision since Medicare began. If one assumes, plausibly, that prospective payment is here to stay, several modifications are likely to be discussed at length in the near future. First, as noted earlier, prospective payment systems might be extended to physicians' services. Second, the government might pass legislation imposing an all-payers system, that is, extending prospective payment systems beyond Medicare to Blue Cross, Medicaid, commercial, and other payers. This would alleviate fears that instead of disciplining themselves to achieve new efficiencies in management and delivery, hospitals will continue their wasteful ways, shifting costs lost on Medicare to other payers. Third, the government might take explicit note of quality problems that may arise from the incentives in prospective payment systems for hospitals to discharge patients "quicker but sicker," thus encouraging readmissions, straining patients' abilities to care for themselves, or depleting the resources of home-health and community-based agencies. In July 1985 Senator John Heinz, Republican of Pennsylvania, chairman of the Special Senate Committee on Aging, charged that in "several thousand" cases Medicare patients had been discharged too fast or transferred inappropriately, and in several cases had died as a result. Heinz contended that the peer review organizations, supposedly watchdogs over the quality of care in Medicare, "appear to be paralyzed," in part for want of clear instructions from the Department of Health and Human Services on their duties.[74] Fourth, to achieve equity among institutions, the diagnosis-related group-based system may need modification. The most prominent recommendation is that a "severity index" be incorporated into the payment mechanism to ensure that hospitals that treat patients whose conditions are more complicated than the diagnosis-related groups acknowledge will not be penalized.[75] Fifth, the government might consider approaches to prospective payment systems other than diagnosis-related groups. Perhaps fee schedules negotiated between payers (public, private, or both) and providers (organizations of hospitals and physicians) are preferable. Or perhaps global budgeting is a more reliable means of cost-containment than such per-case payments as diagnosis-related groups. Or perhaps capitation—a fixed amount paid per unit of time for the care of each beneficiary—is the form of prospective payment most suited to contain costs.[76]

Option 4. The federal government could try finally to devise an area-based planning system with the capacity and power to relate needs to resources. Planning, currently the weakest regulatory tool, may also be the linchpin of a coherent regulatory system. Rate setting can help curb excessive increases in the unit prices of services but by itself can do little about the mix of services and facilities, so crucial to volume and therefore to cost. Controls on service mix and facilities generally mean utilization review and capital expenditure review respectively, but each should be viewed in the context of the other, and a desirable blend of services, facilities, and rates should reflect the properties of the populations of defined geographical areas—localities, regions, states. Thus the perpetual challenge to devise a planning structure that is neither enfeebled by giving too weak a voice to payers (as were the Health Systems Agencies) nor overwhelmed by their concerns at the expense of weakly represented interests, a structure sufficiently independent of the parochial interests of localities and providers to address the larger public interest but not so technocratic and bureaucratic as to lack political accountability.

Conclusions

The deep involvement of the American federal government in the health-care system is, by comparative standards, of very recent vintage. Belatedly shaking off a long history of deference to private, state, and local prerogatives, the federal government has assumed a significant role in health care only since 1945, a sizable role only since 1965. But in this time, and especially during the last fifteen years, the policy process has telescoped an evolutionary pattern broadly similar to what one finds in other comparable nations.

In essence this policy evolution comprises two periods, the first encompassing twenty to twenty-five years (depending on how one interprets the ambiguous years, 1965-1970) marked by rising concern to redress inequities, growing acceptance of a larger role for the public sector in the health-care system, and a new faith in the central government in particular. This was a period of "breakthrough" politics, in which debate focused on the wisdom of adding new commitments to the federal agenda. These politics generated the major subsidy programs that supported providers in building the system's capacity and the financing entitlements that built new access to that system among consumers. Equity was the heart of the period's public philosophy.

This breakthrough era was followed by fifteen to twenty years dominated by the conviction that the policy system had become overloaded by public and private participants afflicted with "interest-group liberalism" and other such pathologies, a sense of stagnation and loss of purpose and coherence in federal policy, and a movement toward "rationalizing" politics in which debate concentrated on repairing what was already on the federal agenda without making major new additions to it. From these debates came reorganizational efforts, which tried to improve policy and contain costs by a market-oriented strategy, and regulatory programs, which sought to build new governmental controls into the system. Efficiency had become the order of the day.

This compressed policy development shows some important parallels with comparable nations. European nations, too, especially those on the Continent, enthusiastically enlarged their supply of hospitals, physicians, and technology, and they, too, are plagued by surpluses and the high costs they entail. In Europe, too, third parties pay for most medical care, and health insurance costs are said to be increasingly insupportable. In Europe broader benefits are balanced by tighter controls; in the United States smaller benefits are offset by weaker controls, so the two reach a similar expensive outcome by dissimilar routes. European nations also ponder the possibility of enlisting reorganization and regulation in the cost-containment cause and even admire, at least in

theory, the HMOs, PPOs, DRGs, PSROs, and other alphabetical prog-
eny of our fevered organizational imagination.

In other respects, however—particularly in the financing arena—
European and American cultures and practices remain distinct. Europe
has built national health insurance on a universal consensus that health
care is a right. The United States has built "national" health insurance
mainly on work-related health insurance in the private sector, leaving a
gap-filling role for government, and no coverage at all for 10 percent to
15 percent of the population. In the United States health care is a fringe
benefit for most of the population, an entitlement qualified by categorical criteria for many, a matter of chance and charity for some. And,
whatever Europeans' fascination with American innovations in reorganization and regulation, they are inclined to pursue cost-containment
by negotiations over the details of fees schedules or the allocation of
global budgets among payers and providers in corporatist settings, an
approach that is alien to American practice but one that may be gradually finding its place in functional substitutes here, too.[77]

In their incomplete convergence with European patterns, American
health-care policies illuminate basic dilemmas of the American welfare
state. Whatever its specific form, the welfare state, American or other,
rests on two fundamental supports. The first, which may be termed
moral or categorical (as in "categorical imperative"), maintains that it
is simply wrong for society to allow some of its citizenry to go without
income, decent housing, food, schooling, work, and health services.
The second foundation, which is practical or utilitarian, holds that redistributive measures to assist the vulnerable help keep the social fabric
intact ("regulating the poor"). Dogmatists to the contrary, neither variation is alone sufficient to explain the politics of the modern welfare state;
both values and interests invariably play their part and deserve their due.
But their roles differ in strength and in relative importance; in the United
States both foundations are relatively weak.

Today social Darwinists are hard to find and everyone believes in the
safety net, but we retain an astonishing ability to ignore holes in it—for
example, a degree of rationing of medical care by price that appalls
European observers. The most plausible explanation is not merely
moral indifference but rather a latent empirical assumption that rationing by price is backstopped and mitigated by rationing by chance; that
is, the medically indigent can show up at the emergency room or outpa-

tient clinic of a hospital, probably will be treated, and will be written off as a charity case or bad debt, ultimately showing up in everyone's insurance premiums or tax bills. Thus, no one must go utterly without care after all; and is this solution not preferable to all the controversies and costs of national health insurance, especially when one cannot be entirely sure that the disadvantaged in question are truly deserving, given that (a fortiori) they have not qualified for Medicare or Medicaid? Nor are Americans wholly without concern for the social fabric; indeed, we engage in flamboyant policy gymnastics when it is stretched, as in the 1960s. Still, for a variety of familiar reasons—the absence of strong leftist political parties, the traditional ambivalence of important elements of the labor movement toward the welfare state, the heterogeneity and lack of organization of those lacking health insurance, ethnic divisions among the poor, the fragmenting force of federalism—it is rarely necessary to "regulate" the disadvantaged by means of public programs.

Given the comparative weakness of the moral and practical foundations of the American welfare state, one would expect to find programs difficult to enact, relatively small in scope and cost, and subject to intermittent challenge. Housing programs conform to the expectation, having evolved over fifty years from a largely unmet commitment to public housing, to a set of subsidies to the private sector to spur construction of rental and single-family units, to retrenchment and vouchers. Many other programs, however, have achieved surprising stability by grasping the secret of success in the politics of the American welfare state, namely, cultivating constituencies beyond their immediate beneficiaries. Welfare programs, for instance, appeal to the intergovernmental lobby of states, counties, and localities, and education draws on the support of the states, localities, and organized teachers. The health-care programs have learned this lesson too. Medicare draws strength from the powerful nexus of labor, liberals, and the elderly that protects Social Security, and Medicaid gains support from the diverse groups that protect federal public assistance programs as well as from health providers. In this way the health-financing programs, along with the social insurance system, public assistance, and unemployment compensation, have become pillars of the American welfare state. Furthermore, the subsidy programs enjoy strong support among providers, and the reorganization and regulatory programs appeal to payers. Over the past forty years, then, the four arenas of federal health-care policy have contrived to offer something to almost everyone—providers, consumers, payers—and have as a result achieved considerable stability. Clearly, stability has not precluded flexibility, but innovation has by and large meant accumulation, piling new "rationalizing" projects onto existing commitments that are held relatively harmless.

Today federal policy cheerfully embodies programs to enlarge the stock of health-care resources and services and other programs to constrain it, programs to expand access to care and others to contain and rechannel it. In the American setting, welfare-state programs may gain stability by assuming a dual role as producer programs too; a sizable measure of policy inefficiency may be the price of political success. One need not overstate the point. Federal policy has largely stopped supporting new hospital construction, has slashed support for medical training, has begun moving to reduce the supply of foreign medical graduates, has put a temporary freeze on physicians' fees in Medicare, and has imposed some redistribution of dollars among hospitals in the prospective payment system. Retrenchment has been fairly modest so far, however, and one wonders how severely a serious assault on the interests of providers and payers might damage programs that probably could not survive easily on the political strength and legitimacy of their beneficiaries alone.

The intricate and perhaps inevitable connection between political stability and policy inefficiency means, among other things, that more and more welfare-state dollars flow into the health sector over time. The costs of growth-as-usual are, first, that the existing configuration of programs is enlarged at the expense of true innovation (because Medicare spends so much fulfilling the "medical model," there is no money for new long-term-care benefits based on home and community-based models; because Medicaid pays so much to hospitals and nursing homes there are few "extra" funds for pre- and postnatal-care benefits) and, second, that money is withheld from other worthy activities (some welfare-state in character, some not) such as housing, environmental protection, higher income supports, educational programs, manpower training, nutrition, and others. Some critics of the welfare state would happily accept at least the second cost, arguing that these latter programs are, by and large, Great Society enthusiasms that failed—a charge that could be upheld to some degree for some programs, very

little for others, and in any case cannot be pursued here. It is hard to
defend an a priori verdict that these other claims cannot be honored
because legal and political entitlements vested in health care's medical
model are sacrosanct.

The dilemma is obvious and eternal. So much needs doing in the
health field even as the growth of health costs diverts scarce resources
from other fields in which there is also so much to be done. In theory the
dilemma is easily dispelled. Rational policies would, first, slow the flow
of dollars into the health-care system, diverting savings to other worthy
areas, and, second, redistribute those smaller funds within the health
sector in ways that reduce waste and target need so that no one goes
without and new benefits are sustainable. But in practice we know, first,
that money saved on the health budget may go to the Strategic Defense
Initiative (Star Wars), not child nutrition, and, second, that redistribution within the health sector may harm, not help, the disadvantaged.
And so one defends the national health-care budget with an increasingly
uneasy conscience.

The political realities seem to augur poorly for equity and for those
who would see the federal role in health care come closer to the philo-
sophical heart of the welfare state by focusing on society's most vulnerable members. To be sure, the heyday of concern for equity has long
since (that is, since 1970) given way to a preoccupation with efficiency,
but the relation between the two may prove to be dialectical after all.
The political history of the breakthroughs of the 1940s, 1950s, and
1960s shows a myopic if laudable focus on equity that sowed the seeds
of the efficiency-mindedness to come. The unconstrained introduction
and diffusion of technology, excess hospital beds, the physician surplus, the retrospective cost-based reimbursement system, and the
assignment of the cost of long-term care to Medicaid by default were
understandable failures of policy design born of lack of foresight and an
excusable political urge to answer while opportunity briefly knocked.
The system has wrestled with their legacy for a decade and a half.
Today, however, policy makers are pushing efficiency with unprecedented resolve and the policy dialectic may be on the point of reemerg-
ing. Today's policy theme may be summarized (with wanton disregard
for the decent limits of alliteration) as prudent purchasers practicing prospective payment with preferred providers. The prudent purchaser may
be content to shift costs to other imprudent (or benevolent) purchasers

and to "cream off" the better risks. Prospective payment can be designed to eliminate cross-subsidies among payer categories and service units. Preferred providers can enhance their competitive edge by dumping the more complicated cases and the less profitable ill. As these trends accelerate the informal rationing by chance that has long allowed public opinion to blink at the cruelty of rationing by price is breaking down; providers can afford only so much free care before they run their institutions, hard pressed both by prospective payment and competition, into the red. As the distribution of opportunities for free care contracts, the moral cost of rationing by price grows higher and more visible. Conceivably, the outcome will be sufficiently distasteful to return equity to the policy agenda.

If so, it will be seen that the disadvantaged can reliably be cared for only if cross-subsidies are reintroduced and redefined. In essence, there are only two ways of helping those who cannot afford their own care—through insurance premiums (community rating, paying rates set by public authorities to cover subsidies to hospitals, or pooled funding, for example) or through new or higher taxes. And there are only two plausible objects of assistance—needy individuals and the institutions that serve them. In time something must give—either the prudent purchaser must admit a dash of imprudence or new tax dollars must be raised or transferred for this purpose—and something must be given—either new financing entitlements for individuals or new subsidies for providers. In short, by pushing reorganization and regulatory strategies to their logical conclusions, policy makers are reawakening the old equity questions at the heart of the subsidy and financing arenas.

This possibility should not be read as an invitation to unfurl the motheaten banner of national health insurance, still less that of a national health service. The creation of Medicare and Medicaid was, so to speak, an exercise in simple addition: the one was grafted onto Social Security before its "crisis," the other to the welfare system before it had become a "mess," and no one then worried about the excess supply and cost in the medical mainstream to which the new programs were to assure access. Answering the equity questions of the 1980s is a venture into the higher calculus. We have too much on the supply side and know too much about the demand side to accept facile assumptions about the relations among needs, resources, and costs. The challenge, then, is to give both equity and efficiency their simultaneous due in a health system that plays an important but limited role in the larger welfare state. Answering the challenge demands a creative yet realistic arrangement of the pieces of the policy puzzle set forth here. Conservatives may seize upon such options as competition, cost-sharing, state experimentation, and vouchers. Liberals may opt for technology assessment, diagnosis-related group or capitation payment to physicians, long-term-care benefits in Medicare, a federalized Medicaid, capital caps, an all-payers prospective payment system, and stronger planning. But a truly consistent ideological solution is no longer possible. The responsible liberal and conservative will listen and learn, mix and match. There is no correct solution to the puzzle and this paper offers no blueprint. Its sole purpose has been to display some major options for the possible benefit of policy makers, who may understand better than today's prudent purchasers that in politics (as Burke put it) "magnanimity . . . is not seldom the truest wisdom," and that in the welfare state rationality and benevolence may enlighten, not exclude, each other.

Notes and References

1. Adams, H.: *The Education of Henry Adams*. Boston, Houghton Mifflin, 1961, p. 400.

2. Cochrane, A.L.: *Effectiveness and Efficiency: Random Reflections on Health Services*. London, Nuffield Provincial Hospitals Trust, 1972, chap. 8.

3. For an elaboration of this framework see Brown, L.D.: *Politics and Health Care Organization: HMOs as Federal Policy*. Washington, D.C., Brookings Institution, 1983, chap. 1; Brown, L.D.: *New Policies, New Politics: Government's Response to Government's Growth*. Washington, D.C., Brookings Institution, 1983.

4. Goldsmith, J.C.: *Can Hospitals Survive?* Homewood, Ill., Dow Jones–Irwin, 1981, p. 11.

5. Wildavsky, A.: "Doing Better and Feeling Worse: The Political Pathology of Health Policy." In: *Doing Better and Feeling Worse: Health in the United States*, Knowles, J.H., editor. New York, Norton, 1977, p. 122. For a corrosive view of prevention see Stone, D.A., "The Resistible Rise of Preventive Medicine," *J. Health Politics Policy Law 11*: 671-696, 1986.

6. Strickland, S.R.: *U.S. Health Care: What's Wrong and What's Right*. New York, Universe Books, 1972, p. 37.

7. Russell, L.B.: *Technology in Hospitals: Medical Advances and Their Diffusion*. Washington, D.C., Brookings Institution, 1979, pp. 43, 45, 47, 65, 70.

8. See Cochrane's plea for this approach, op. cit., chapters 4, 5.

9. Ruby, G., Banta, H.D., and Burns, A.K.: "Medicare Coverage, Medicare Costs and Medical Technology." *J. Health Politics Policy Law 10*: 141-151, 1985.

10. Cohen, A.B., and Cohodes, D.R.: "Certificate of Need and Low Capital-Cost Medical Technology." *Milbank Mem. Fund Quart. Health Soc. 60*: 320, 1982.

11. Salkever, D.S., and Bice, T.W.: *Hospital Certificate-of-Need Controls: Impact on Investment, Costs, and Use*. Washington, D.C., American Enterprise Institute for Public Policy Research, 1979.

12. Interview with the author.

13. See, for example, the views of a Maryland planner quoted in Brown, L.D.: "Common Sense Meets Implementation: Certificate-of-Need Regulation in the States." *J. Health Politics Policy Law 8*: 485, 1983.

14. Moloney, T.W. and Rogers, D.E.: "Medical Technology—A Different View of the Contentious Debate over Costs." *N. Engl. J. Med. 301*: 1413-1419, 1979.

15. Aaron, H.J., and Schwartz, W.B.: *The Painful Prescription: Rationing Hospital Care*. Washington, D.C., Brookings Institution, 1984, pp. 117-118.

16. Brown, L.D.: "Civil Rights and Regulatory Wrongs: The Reagan Administration and the Medical Treatment of Handicapped Newborns." *J. Health Politics Policy Law 11*: 231-542, 1986.

17. Institute of Medicine: *Controlling the Supply of Hospital Beds: A Policy Statement*. Washington, D.C., National Academy of Sciences, 1976, pp. vii, ix, 2, 7, 15.

18. Department of Health and Human Services: *Health, United States, 1984*. Hyattsville, Md., DHHS Pub. No. (PHS) 85-1232, December 1984, pp. 126, 127, and *Health, United States, 1987*, DHHS Pub. No. (PHS) 88-1232, March 1987, pp. 135, 138.

19. This account of Michigan's effort follows Carpenter, E.S., and Paul-Shaheen, P.: "Implementing Regulatory Reform: The Saga of Michigan's Debedding Experiment." *J. Health Politics Policy Law 9*: 457-460, 462, 469, 1984.

20. Thorpe, K.E.: "Does All-Payer Rate Setting Work? The Case of the New York Prospective Hospital Reimbursement Methodology," *J. Health Politics Policy Law 12*: 391-408, 1987.

21. Vladeck, B.C.: *Unloving Care: The Nursing Home Tragedy*. New York, Basic Books, 1980, pp. 228-229.

22. See Barer, Morris L.: "Regulatory Physician Supply: The Evolution of British Columbia's Bill 41." *J. Health Politics Policy Law 13*: 1-25, 1988.

23. *Summary Report of the Graduate Medical Education National Advisory Committee to the Secretary, Department of Health and Human Services*, vol. 1. Washington, D.C., DHHS Pub. No. (HRA) 81-651, September 30, 1980, pp. 3, 7.

24. Ibid., p. 3; Rimm, A.A.: Letter to editor. *N. Engl. J. Med. 313*: 699, 1985.

25. Iglehart, J.K.: "Health Policy Report: Reducing Residency Opportunities for Graduates of Foreign Medical Schools." *N. Engl. J. Med. 313*: 831-836, quotation at 836, 1985.

26. Hadley, J.: "Physician Supply and Distribution." In: *National Health Insurance: Conflicting Goals and Policy Choices,* Feder, J., et al., editors. Washington, D.C., Urban Institute, 1980, p. 233. For a useful discussion, see Mick, S.S., "Contradictory Policies for FMGs." *Health Affairs 6*: 5-18, 1987.

27. For an overview see GMENAC: *Summary Report*, p. 39.

28. Ebert, R.H., and Ginzberg, E.: "The Reform of Medical Education"; "Perspective: A Representative"; and Jolly, P.: "DataWatch: Medical Education in the United States, 1960-1987" *Health Affairs*: 7:8, 45, 148, 1988.

29. The 20% figure comes from Hadley, op. cit., p. 191; the 30% figure and figures for Europe are from Schroeder, S.A.: "The Making of a Medical Generalist." *Health Affairs 4*: 29, 1985.

30. Schwartz, W.B., et al.: "The Changing Geographic Distribution of Board-Certified Physicians." *N. Engl. J. Med. 303*: 1032-1038, 1980.

31. The term comes from Smith, B.W.H., and Gerard, R.J.: "A Federal Health Service Corps." *N. Engl. J. Med. 306*: 1045, 1982.

32. Hadley, op. cit., p. 237; Smith and Gerard, op. cit., p. 1046.

33. Hadley, ibid., p. 238; Blumenthal, D.: "Right Turns, Wrong Turns and Roads Untaken: The Discretionary Federal Health Budget." In: *Health Care: How to Improve It and Pay for It.* Washington, D.C., Center for National Policy, 1985, p. 68.

34. Jencks, S.F., and Dobson, A.: "Strategies for Reforming Medicare's Physician Payments." *N. Engl. J. Med. 312*: 1492-1499, 1985 (the source of the discussion in this paragraph).

35. Ibid., p. 1495.

36. Mitchell, J.B.: Physicians DRGs. *N. Engl. J. Med. 313*: 670, 1985.

37. Schwartz, W.B., et al: "Why There Will Be Little or No Physician Surplus Between Now and the Year 2000," and Schloss, E.P.: "Beyond GMENAC—Another Physician Shortage from 2010 to 2030?" *N. Engl. J. Med. 318*: 892-897, 920-922, 1988.

38. On the political uses of this argument and the problems with it see Derthick, M.: *Policymaking for Social Security.* Washington, D.C., Brookings Institution, 1979.

39. For the political background see Sundquist, J.L.: *Politics and Policy: The Eisenhower, Kennedy, and Johnson Years.* Washington, D.C., Brookings

Institution, 1968, chap. 7; Marmor, T.R.: *The Politics of Medicare*. Chicago, Aldine, 1973.

40. Rice, D.P., and Feldman, J.J.: "Living longer in the United States: Demographic Changes and Health Needs of the Elderly." *Milbank Mem. Fund Quart. Health Soc. 61*: 362, 372-373, 1983.

41. See ibid., pp. 378-384, for specific projections.

42. "Summary of the 1983 Annual Reports of the Medicare Board of Trustees." *Health Care Financ. Rev. 5*: 2-3, 1983.

43. The figures in this paragraph are taken from DHHS: *Health, United States, 1984*, tables 89 and 91, and from Davis, K.: "Access to Health Care: A Matter of Fairness." In: Center for National Policy: *Health Care*, pp. 47-48.

44. Rice and Feldman, op. cit., pp. 382, 384.

45. The list is taken from Ginsburg, P.B., and Moon, M.: "An Introduction to the Medicare Financing Problem." *Milbank Mem. Fund Quart. Health Soc. 62*: 174-181, 1984.

46. Cited in Marmor, T.R., and Dunham, A.: "The Politics of Health Policy Reform: Problems, Origins, Alternatives, and a Possible Prescription." In: Center for National Policy: *Health Care*, p. 36.

47. Ibid.

48. Ibid., p. 41.

49. Davis, K., and Rowland, D.: "Medicare Financing Reform: A New Medicare Premium." *Milbank Mem. Fund Quart. Health Soc. 62*: 307-308, 1984; Munnell, A.H.: "Enhancing Medicare Revenues." *J. Health Politics Policy Law 10*: 489-511, 1985.

50. Davis and Rowland, op. cit., p. 308; Meyer, J.: "Comment on 'Medicare financing reform: A new Medicare premium,' " pp. 319-320.

51. Munnell, op. cit.

52. Ibid.

53. On the politics and problems of the hospice benefit see Fraser, I.: "Medicare Reimbursement for Hospice Care: Ethical and Policy Implications of Cost Containment Strategies." *J. Health Politics Policy Law 10*: 565-577, 1985.

54. Somers, A.R.: "Long-Term Care for the Elderly and Disabled: An Urgent Challenge to New Federalism." In: *New Federalism and Long-Term Health Care of the Elderly*, Dunlop, B.D., editor. Millwood, Va., Project HOPE, 1985, p. 52.

55. Ibid., p. 91, comments by Richard E. Curtis.

56. Smith, J.I.: "Block Grant Experiences: Illusions and Realities." In: *New*

Federalism and Long-Term Health Care of the Elderly, pp. 63-70.

57. Somers, "Long-Term Care."op. cit., pp. 56-57.

58. Davidson, J.: "U.S. Study Cites Distressing Disparity in Health Conditions for Blacks, Whites." *The Wall Street Journal*, October 15, 1985, p. 12.

59. Haggerty, R.J.: Editorial. "The Limits of Medical Care." *N. Engl. J. Med.* *313*: 383-384, 1985.

60. See Iglehart, J.K.: "Health Policy Report: Medical Care for the Poor—A Growing Problem." *N. Engl. J. Med. 313*: 59-63, 1985; *State Health Notes*, No. 48: 1-3, 1984. Also useful is the state-by-state survey of developments in Federation of American Hospitals: *Review 18*: 20-31, 1985.

61. For some of the reasons see Brown, *Politics and Health Care Organization*.

62. American Medical Care and Review Association Institute for International Health Initiatives: *Directory of Preferred Provider Organizations*. Bethesda, Md., Institute for International Health Initiatives, 1984, p. 2.

63. Figures supplied in June 1988 by S.E. Pickens, Director of Special Projects, American Medical Care and Review Association, Bethesda, Md.

64. For a review of the evidence see Luft, H.S.: *Health Maintenance Organizations: Dimensions of Performance*. New York, Wiley, 1981.

65. Derived from InterStudy: *National HMO Census, 1983*, Excelsior, Minn., InterStudy, 1984, and InterStudy, *The InterStudy Edge: Quarterly Report of HMO Growth and Enrollment as of September 30, 1987*, Excelsior, Minn., InterStudy, 1987.

66. Quotations from Luft, H.S., Maerki, S.C., and Trauner, J.B.: "The Competitive Effects of Health Maintenance Organizations: Another Look at the Evidence from Hawaii, Rochester, and Minneapolis/St. Paul," pp. 625-658, quotation at 654; Johnson, A.N., and Aquilina, D.: "The Competitive Impact of Health Maintenance Organizations and Competition on Hospitals in Minneapolis/St. Paul," pp. 659-674, quotations at 659, 670; Feldman, R., et al.: "The Competitive Impact of Health Maintenance Organizations on Hospital Finances: An Exploratory Study," pp. 675-697, especially 693; and Merrill, J., and McLaughlin, C.: "Competition Versus Regulation: Some Emperical Evidence," pp. 613-623, quotation at 621. *J. Health Politics Policy Law* 10: 1986.

67. This account follows Staver, S.: "Seniors Shut Out of New HMO Program." *Am. Med. News*, pp. 1, 9, June 21, 1985.

68. A helpful review of four programs is Freund, D.A., et al.: *Medicaid Reform: Four Studies of Case Management*. Washington, D.C., American Enterprise Institute for Public Policy Research, 1984. On the theory and practice of the Arizona Health Care Cost Containment System (AHCCS),

see Brecher, C.: "Medicaid Comes to Arizona: A First-Year Report on AHCCS," and Hillman, D.G., and Christianson, J.B.: "Competitive Bidding as a Cost-Containment Strategy for Indigent Medical Care: The Implementation Experience in Arizona." *J. Health Politics Policy Law 9*: 411-451, 1984.

69. Reinhardt, U.: "The Problem of 'Uncompensated Care,' or are Americans Really as Mean as They Look?" In: *Proceedings—Uncompensated Care in a Competitive Environment: Whose Problem Is It?* September 13-14, 1984, HRP-0906304, Washington, D.C.: U.S. Department of Health and Human Services, p. 20.

70. Enthoven, A.: *Health Plan*. Reading, Mass., Addison-Wesley, 1980.

71. See Altman, Stuart H., and Rodwin, Marc A.: "Halfway Competitive Markets and Ineffective Regulation: The American Health Care System," *J. Health Politics Policy Law* 13: 323-339, 1988.

72. For a useful overview, see Eby, C.L., and Cohodes, D.R.: "What Do We Know about Rate-Setting?" *J. Health Politics Policy Law, 10*: 299-327, 1985.

73. On considerations of design, see Brown, L.D.: "Political Conditions of Regulatory Effectiveness: The Case of PSROs and HSAs." *Bull. N. Y. Acad. Med. 58*: 77-90, 1982.

74. United States Senate, Special Committee on Aging: Aging Reports. Washington, D.C., Govt. Print. Off., 1985, pp. 1, 3.

75. Horn, S.D., et al.: "Interhospital Differences in Severity of Illness." *N. Engl. J. Med. 313*: 20-24, 1985.

76. For a wide-ranging and instructive review of European practice see Glaser, W.A.: *Paying the Hospital*. San Francisco, Jossey-Bass, 1987.

77. On these and related issues, see Marmor, Theodore R.: "American Medical Policy and the 'Crisis' of the Welfare State: A Comparative Perspective," *J. Health Politics Policy Law 11*: 617-631, 1986. Also, Starr, Paul, and Immergut, Ellen: "Health Care and the Boundaries of Politics." In: Maier, Charles, S.: *Changing Boundaries of the Political: Essays on the Evolving Balance Between the State and Society, Public and Private, in Europe*. Cambridge, Cambridge University Press, 1987, pp 221-254.